Getting
Your
Second
Wind

Blessings on your path to wellness!
Jan

Jan Tilley

Getting Your Second Wind

Published by Wheatmark®
610 East Delano Street, Suite 104
Tucson, Arizona 85705 U.S.A.
www.wheatmark.com

International Standard Book Number: 978-1-60494-133-3
Library of Congress Control Number: 2008928903

To my beautiful children, Leigh, Tabette, Lindsey and Jay, who have stood beside me through good times and bad. Each of you in your own amazing way have taught me courage and strength, and have given me more joy than I ever thought possible.

To my mom, Ganelle, who has loved me unconditionally and has modeled for me the secret to aging gracefully. Mom, your spirit and your passion for living are my inspiration.

To my husband, Bruce, you encourage me to greatness in everything I do. You believe in me and support my passion for living life to the fullest. Thank you for loving me so completely.

To my father, Jack, who lived a life of passion. Dad, I inherited that burning need you had to experience all that life has to offer AND the strong calling you had to go out and make a difference in the world. We are so much alike and I miss you terribly. I wish you were here to see that I am still striving and reaching for more, but, through the grace of God, I have found joy and peace in the process.

Contents

Introduction

Have you taken a good look at yourself lately and wondered, "How did I let myself get in this shape?" Does each passing year leave you lugging around additional weight?

Is your energy lagging? Have the challenges of everyday life drained the passion, fun, and excitement from you? Is it time for a fresh start?

The human spirit is amazing in that it seeks balance. When life gets off course, and it seems everything is spiraling out of control, a fighting spirit exists within each of us driving us to get back on track. We must allow that inner drive to motivate us to take action. If we squelch the desire, we run the risk of becoming complacent and settling for less than the best in life. If we embrace the opportunity to make changes, we are able to grow and become all God has created us to be.

Life is a journey we all are privileged to take. It is filled with joy, sorrow, and challenge. Some of this arrives through no one's fault; some is brought on by choice. In either case, we have the opportunity to choose our response.

Many have chosen to follow a path-of-least-resistance approach to life. They have adopted a lifestyle of poor eating habits and nonexistent fitness goals. Choosing this lifestyle will age you far beyond your years. It can lead to a life of obesity and a challenge-filled aging process plagued with joint problems, diabetes, heart disease, hypertension, and cancer.

Others have chosen to live a healthy, active life. These are people who look and act younger than their years. This group will likely avoid many challenges associated with aging. They may stay competitive in sports, be able to jump on the floor to play with the grandkids, and continue an active, vibrant life well into their later years.

I have a nutrition and fitness practice where I teach clients to eat healthy and develop fit bodies. I see the pain of growing old without health and fitness and, believe me, it's not a pretty sight. However, this is a book designed to tell you more than how to lose weight and stay fit.

I believe three essential components are keys to healthy living. We will never reach our full potential without all three. Our physical bodies need to be properly nourished and trained. Our mental capacity needs to be challenged with tasks that allow us to grow and develop. As important as those two are, there is a third component I believe to be paramount in allowing us to navigate a successful journey through life—a positive, joyful attitude. I've seen it make a difference over and over again in my own life and in the lives of my clients, my family, and my friends.

Joy is found by choosing to focus on the good aspects of life and accepting or being content with the difficult things in life that cannot be changed. It is a mental shift where we look at our circumstances differently. We see them for what they can teach us and how they can help us grow. By learning to reposition our approach, we make peace with our situation. We are able to catch our breath, find our second wind, and run the race of life with newfound strength, courage, and grace.

Now, if you are wondering how you can be joyful despite all you might be going through, let me share my observations with you. Many of the people who exude true joy have, in reality, had a difficult life. The key to their overcoming adversity is their willingness to embrace the journey. To them, life is an adventure intended to sharpen and refine the character of those who actively participate in it. Those who choose joy have learned to savor the good, learn from the bad, and embrace the daily challenges that come their way as another opportunity for personal growth. After all, a joyous life is not something that just happens to you; it is a choice that results from a grateful heart.

It's funny how we learn some of our life lessons. After my brother and I were grown and gone from home, my parents became missionaries in Panama. During a visit to see them, we attended a Sunday evening service in Colon, Panama. The congregation was primarily Panamanian nationals who lived in the impoverished inner city of Colon. I distinctly remember meeting this strikingly beautiful, chocolate-skinned woman in a perfectly starched white dress. Her name was Gloria, and she had her young son with her. I learned from my mom that Gloria earned her living cleaning houses. The memorable thing about her was her smile. It made such an impression on me because I was in a difficult place in my life—single mom of four young children struggling to make ends meet—and I was feeling sorry for myself.

My life's burden felt heavy, and my joy was definitely in short supply. After the service, I had the opportunity to visit with her and as we talked, she said, "I am blessed beyond measure." I'm thinking to myself, she walks to and from work each day. She lives in a tiny apartment above an open-air market in a dangerous inner city. Yet, I could tell she sincerely felt blessed. Her face glowed and her smile was a great reminder of all I had to be thankful for. Gloria provided a powerful demonstration of the chosen joy born out of a grateful heart.

The inspiration to make life changes often comes to you through little unexpected moments such as this. I could see in Gloria something lacking in my own life, and I knew it was time to put my life in order.

This book is about fresh starts. If you have taken some wrong turns and ended up in a place you never wanted or intended to be, this book's message is for you. It is about beginning again. Whether you are young, old or somewhere in between. If life has thrown you for a loop, it is time to get up, dust yourself off, and start down a path leading to a life of health and purpose.

This book is my story—the good, the bad and the ugly. I am sharing it with you to demonstrate God has proven to be my patient, faithful companion, even when I have chosen to do things my own way. He has been a gentleman, allowing me the freedom to try and fail. He has stood beside me through thick and thin and has taught me that I can quit pretending. He loves me for exactly who I am. He has seen my heart and has chosen to use me in spite of my flaws. He has taken my night and turned it to day. He is the joy of my life.

It is my hope that in some small way, my story will resonate with you and encourage you to make practical life changes that allow you to grow into the life you desire. No magic. Just a straightforward approach to choosing your way to health and joy. Let the journey begin.

Foreword

I was sitting in the Cooper Clinic in Dallas, Texas, when I first heard the words that prompted me to reconsider the choices I was making in my life. Dr. Kenneth Cooper, the renowned physician and author, was the speaker, and these were the words: "We should all strive to live a long and active life followed by an exceedingly short death." It is so true, yet as I sat there contemplating the statement, I was convicted by the poor choices I had made regarding my well-being. At that very moment—the instant I thought this—it hit me: I was not fit to lead ... or get the most out of my life physically, mentally, or spiritually.

I have always been a student of history, but when it comes to my own past, I have a healthy disdain for times gone by. Perhaps like you, my history was full of mistakes— my life journey seemed to be one poor choice after another. For many years, I shouldered the burden of guilt and the pain of disappointment on my own. I countered my depression by eating foods based solely on their emotional appeal, not their nutritional value. As the days turned into weeks and the weeks into months, even years, my effectiveness as a leader, a husband, a father, and a friend was impacted negatively.

Rather than seek help, I did what most men do: I fought it. And, when I failed (which was often) I beat myself up. It was my selfish way of ensuring a life marked by remorse and regret. After all, I had no right to be joyful—I was paying the price for my poor choices, each and every day. Oh, I suppose from a distance I appeared to have it all together. I had a good job, money in the bank, a loving family, and a church membership. Sadly, though, I was a broken soul. In fact, as I reflect on those days, I now see the way my pride prevented me from enjoying life. Perhaps this is the first lesson of Jan Tilley's wonderful book: Life is meant to be enjoyed.

Like Jan, at some point (after trying to deal with everything by myself) I surrendered to God. I simply could not go on. I longed for the joy of Christianity—the peace embraced by the apostle Paul, among others, throughout New Testament scripture. In retrospect, I am embarrassed to admit it: Despite my own public confession of faith, I was living each day without truly understanding the meaning of the Cross.

Even so, I took my place each Sunday morning alongside hundreds of others, worshipping my Lord and Savior. Like so many people today, I was going through the motions without really understanding the magnitude of the message. I felt hopeless. My well-being (physical, mental, and spiritual) was slipping away. I feared the future.

Max Lucado, the gifted Christian author, would suggest I was dragging a lot of sin-filled baggage along for the journey—my yoke was heavy. I was weighed down by the luggage of life. Max had it right when he penned *Traveling Light* in 2001. In describing history's most beautiful and most horrible moment, Lucado wrote, "Jesus stood in the tribunal of heaven. Sweeping a hand over all creation, he pleaded, 'Punish me for their mistakes. See the murderer? Give me his penalty. The adulteress? I'll take her shame. The bigot, the liar, the thief? Do to me what you would do to them. Treat me as you would a sinner.' And God did."

Like so many people today, I was busy grading my sin each night before bedtime. Inherent in the process was the ever-present temptation to compare my sin with the sins I perceived others committing. I was doing nothing more than rationalizing my behavior in hopes of justifying my salvation before God. Today, it sounds harsh to suggest, but I think a shocking number of adults—many who appear to have it all—are in the same predicament. We fool ourselves into believing that somehow sin can be managed like a checkbook or a calendar. When things get out of sorts, we often turn to destructive things to feel better about ourselves or we simply deposit a few good deeds or insert some time for compassion into our busy schedules, as if such changes will eliminate our shame.

However, life's luggage is not so easily packed away. Sadly, our sins deliver an overwhelming portion of guilt that eats its way through our bodies from the inside out, and no amount of money, sex, or drugs will stop the pain. Whether our sins are loud enough for everyone to see or so quiet that only we know of their existence, no joy can be found in this process; only remorse and regret dwell here. I am convinced God does not want it to be this way. Another life is there for us to live—one full of eternal joy—but we must choose to embrace it.

Getting your Second Wind begins with acknowledging that what happened on the Cross was enough to bring all mankind to God, the righteous and the unrighteous. In other words, God's only son, Jesus Christ, died on the Cross once for all. It is done. It is complete. So what now is our response?

We place our suitcases of mistakes, our satchels of disappointment, and our hanging bags of imperfection at the foot of the Cross, for God's grace is sufficient for those who seek Him. This is the wellspring of our joy.

Here. Now. This very instant, let us all Get our Second Wind, not because of what we have done, but because of what He has done.

For where we are not perfect, He is perfect. For where we have faults, He is faultless. To deny God's remarkable plan is to trivialize the power of the Cross—and, in doing so, concede the only true source of lasting joy. This is the compelling message at the heart of Jan Tilley's inspiring story.

God understands this. He knows life is largely about self-discovery. He knows the fabric of our lives for He is constantly weaving the threads into one amazing tapestry. He blends the people and places that exist in our lives into a colorful image that ultimately represents our unique character. Without the blood of Christ, the tapestry would reveal an assortment of imperfect threads—nothing more than an eyesore with little value.

But, with the blood of Christ, the tapestry reveals a beautiful image—a priceless work of art unlike any other. This is the image God has of his children, and this is the joy that surpasses all understanding. For this reason, we genuinely strive each day to marry our faith to our faithfulness. It is hard, but still we try.

As you read Jan's book, I think you will agree with me—it is a moving testimonial. As a published author, I understand the transformation that occurs during the writing of a book this personal. Like the Sunday school teacher preparing for class, the author of a work such as this most often proves to be the greatest beneficiary. It cleanses the soul and rekindles the hope for a better tomorrow. Jan's life, like every life, reflects a journey of self-discovery. Despite enormous vulnerability, Jan takes us inside her private life, through the painful process of divorce, a harrowing experience with a daughter's eating disorder, and the deep-seated grief caused by the loss of a parent. In doing so, Jan exposes her soul for all to see, and she reminds us all that sometimes we cannot fully appreciate the light seen from the highest summit until we have struggled through the darkness of the deepest valleys.

Such a revelation is not by design—at least not by the author. But this is what happens when we surrender our pride and, as Jan so aptly says, "We choose to be real," because healing can come only after brokenness. Then, we as human beings begin to realize God's plan for us. In Jan's case, it is apparent her message is not really her message at all, but God's message being transmitted through her mind and fingers. As you know, this is how God works. He takes ordinary people and creates extraordinary results.

Getting your Second Wind conveys an extraordinary lesson that provides hope for us all regarding life's journey. From finding the answers to the "big questions" to simply learning how to focus on the smallest blessings each day, Jan does a wonderful job of providing hope to the reader. But this book is so much more. It contains practical solutions for people desiring to make the most out of their lives, physically, mentally, and spiritually.

As I read this manuscript, I was reminded of John F. Kennedy's wise saying, "Change is the law of life. And those who look only to the past or present are certain to miss the future." Getting your Second Wind is Jan's way of urging us to create the future, not miss it.

What a glorious idea: Tomorrow can be better than today.

It starts with a genuine desire to choose wisely. Jan has provided a system we can apply immediately to build a solid foundation for living. Together, each of us can create a bright future by choosing to exercise, choosing to eat right, and choosing to follow God's plan for our lives.

These are not small choices. They are, in fact, the choices that will define our well-being.

How will our character be molded to reflect Christ? What will the impact be on the threads of people and places God is weaving into our lives? Will our lives reflect joy or will our lives reflect baggage and guilt? Will we live long and active lives, followed by exceedingly short deaths? As we contemplate these questions, let us be reminded of Jan's advice:

1. Open your eyes to life's simple pleasures.

2. Open your heart to find your passion.

3. Choose to get in the game.

4. Stretch yourself.

5. Never give up.

Getting your Second Wind provides the encouragement to begin a new journey.

So what now?

Let us Get our Second Wind.

DAN J. SANDERS
Author of Built to Serve and
coauthor of Equipped to Lead

Preface

The American Council on Exercise describes "second wind" as the shift over to aerobic metabolism that occurs after the first few minutes of vigorous exercise. As you begin an aerobic workout, you'll feel somewhat out of breath, and your muscles may ache. Your body isn't able to transport oxygen to the active muscles quickly enough so your muscles burn carbohydrate anaerobically, causing an increase in lactic acid production. The more fit you become, the more quickly your body will make the transition back to aerobic metabolism, which is where we get the term "getting your second wind." When you reach this aerobic steady state, you can maintain your stride for an extended duration.

We can apply this same "second wind" scenario to life. Getting Your Second Wind occurs when you are able to work through trials and struggles to find your stride. Once you have made the transition from a hectic, REACTIVE life to a steady, PROACTIVE pace, you will know the peace and joy that come from catching your breath and making a fresh start.

Many of us have experienced the painful existence that occurs when we are out of sync. This can arise as a result of poor choices we've made that have landed us in a place of despair, or from life circumstances that come out of nowhere to knock the wind out of our sails.

I have faced this challenge in my own life and know first-hand the struggles associated with being unable to catch my breath. I now counsel people in my nutrition practice who are searching for the courage and direction to breathe strong and sure once again.

When I began my business, I defined my purpose to be "helping people discover healthy living through nutrition and fitness." I have kept that mission statement, but I have added to it a third component. Originally, I spent countless hours preparing diet and fitness plans to share with my clients. What I soon discovered is this: People who abuse food (either through overeating or undereating) are hurting. They are suffering from some past pain that led them to mistreat their own bodies, or they are experiencing some current pain that has caused them to lose interest in taking care of their body. In either case, they have lost their motivation and the direction they need to get back to a healthy lifestyle. These people don't need my diet plans; they need a personal path to wellness.

Let me further explain by telling you about Belinda. She is 60 years old, 5-foot-5, 285 pounds. She has been on every diet known to man, numerous times throughout her adult life. She usually loses about 30 to 50 pounds, and then gains it all back, plus a few more for good measure. As we talked, I learned that she had a son who was born with a disability. Shortly after that, her marriage fell apart and she cared for her son until he passed away at age 18. She lives alone in a small town in rural South Texas. She sleeps a lot and said she would prefer to sleep 24 hours a day. She has a couple of things that motivate her to get out of bed: She works part-time and attends church Sunday mornings.

In my early years of business, my goal would have been to put Belinda on a low-calorie meal plan and a fitness plan to facilitate a 1 ½- to 2-pound weight loss each week. While I still do this with my clients, my focus is less about helping Belinda lose weight and more about helping her find her "second wind." At our first session, we discussed ideas for how she might find an activity, a group, or a cause that will fuel her passion. This will do more to energize her and build her confidence than all the diet plans I could give her. My job is to help her find a way to turn her hopelessness and despair into passion and purpose. When she does that, she will find the confidence she needs to successfully adopt a healthier lifestyle ... for life.

Taking charge of your life is not easy. It requires good solid direction and a great deal of focus and determination to make it happen. I've written *Getting Your Second Wind* to help encourage you and help illuminate the path by sharing stories from my own life as well as the lives of some of the wonderful people I have been blessed to know.

Those who have successfully discovered their own path to wellness share some common characteristics. In this book, I have selected traits I believe to be instrumental in the process of reinventing yourself to enjoy a life of purpose. I've built a chapter around each characteristic. The first trait is learning to take charge of your life by being open to adventure. You know the old saying, "If you keep doing the same thing, you will keep getting the same result." I challenge you to step to the far edge of your comfort zone. Look out across the wide expanse of possibility. Read these next eleven chapters with a willing heart, wide open to experiencing the amazing life God has planned for you.

CHAPTER I

Take Charge of Your Life:
Be Adventurous

*Being adventurous means learning to live with your
    eyes and your heart wide open to challenge and
    adventure.*
*It means embracing the real you—your passions, your
    talents, your strengths, and your weaknesses.*
*It is finding the courage to take a chance on
    yourself—to become all that you were created for.*

It was a cold January morning in 1985. My children and
I were among a large group of family and friends gathered
at the airport in Lubbock, Texas, to send my parents off to
the war-torn country of Panama during the corrupt reign of
President Manuel Noriega.

For as long as I remember, my parents have had a huge
heart for missions. They took several shorter mission trips to
faraway places while my brother and I were growing up, but
once we were both off on our own, they decided to pull up
their roots in the states and move to a remote location to tell
people about Jesus.

I know making the move must have been a difficult decision. I'm sure they were apprehensive about moving off into the unknown. I know they were sad about leaving behind their elderly parents, my brother and I, and especially their precious grandkids, but even through their sadness you could not miss the sparkle in their eyes. I love the fact that my parents modeled for me a keen sense of adventure. They were passionate and were not afraid to take chances.

I inherited my parent's zest for adventure. I love the thrill that comes from new experiences—sometimes to a fault. My husband is a financial adviser. Everything he does, both at home and at work, involves taking calculated risks. He loves to tease me about the fact that I am very good at taking risks, but I somehow missed the calculated part. He is referring to the fact that I've been known to act first and think it through later. I prefer to think of it as being fun and spontaneous.

In high school, I attended a church youth trip to Lake Fryer near Perryton, Texas, where a large group of us spent the day water skiing and enjoying the lake. Near the end of the day, my best friend, Denise, and I decided to walk across the dam. The lake was low and not flowing over the dam, but ski boats speeding by caused some water to cascade over the dam, leaving gooey, mossy patches.

Always up for a challenge, I convinced Denise to walk with me across the slippery dam. We made it across to the ledge and were coming back, holding on to each other, giggling hysterically and showing off to our friends, who by this time had gathered along the banks to watch us.

Just when we thought we had it made, we slipped and fell into the awful, stagnant, murky water below. It was slimy and we couldn't get a grip on anything to get out. Luckily, we looked up to the rim of the canyon to see a local Boy Scout troop hiking by. They heard the commotion and came to our rescue. They threw us a rope and hoisted us to safety. We escaped unharmed, although our swimsuits were slightly tattered and our arms, legs, and egos were badly bruised.

Isn't that how life is? We're rocking along having a good time. All of a sudden, we make a couple of bad decisions and find ourselves at the bottom of a murky, slimy dam with nothing to grab to pull ourselves back to safety.

As you begin your quest to take charge of your life, you may be just beginning to feel the slippery moss beneath your feet, or you may find that you have slipped so far off course that you have hit rock bottom. The desire to get your second wind can come as the result of catastrophe or complacency. Sometimes our choices have left us in a place of despair and sometimes we have just chosen a life so safe that we long for excitement and adventure. Either way, making a fresh start requires courage and a willingness to take some calculated chances that will help springboard you into the life you long for.

Here's the payoff for stepping out of your comfort zone to try something new: It allows you the mental and physical freedom to experience the wonderful things life has to offer that you might otherwise completely miss. From the time I was old enough to remember, my father instilled within me the confidence to believe I could do and become anything. As a very young girl, I remember saying to him, "Even president of the United States?" and his answer was always, "Yes, even president of the United States. You are smart, you are beautiful, and you can become anything you want to be."

My dad inspired me to greatness. His words continue to be a powerful motivator in my life. His words of confidence were genuine. He loved and believed in me completely. Regardless of any of the awkward stages I went through growing up, I could always hear his words of affirmation. I knew in my heart I was beautiful and capable because my dad told me so.

In all of our lives, obstacles and challenges will inevitably come our way. Facing and overcoming difficulties is what makes us stronger. An easy life (while it seems tempting) does not guarantee a successful life. In nature, the strongest, most resilient plants are those that endure stress and are forced to grow deep roots. These are the plants that grow strong and tall. They overcome hardships to become the best they can be. Likewise, God calls us to be "overcomers" in our lives. Situations and circumstances will trip us and cause us to stumble. Those who determine to take charge of their destiny understand being knocked down and staying down is not an option. We are empowered to steer the direction of our lives.

> *Life ebbs and flows, but through it all, we have a choice to make:*
> *How will we play the cards we are dealt?*
> *Will we allow ourselves to be tossed around by people and circumstances that come our way, or will we take charge of our destiny?*

Several years ago, I found myself dealing with these questions. I had a choice to make. Would I allow circumstances to determine the outcome of my life, or would I take responsibility for myself and embrace the opportunity to become all God created me to be?

As many of you have experienced, once you get moving in a certain direction, it is difficult to change your course. I went through a great deal of internal struggle to get to the point where I was ready to deal with the consequences of taking a new path. For me, deciding to go back to school was the day I "drew a line in the sand" and made the decision to reclaim my life and take it in a different direction. I had been a stay-at-home mom while my children were young, but as I began to come to grips with the fact that my marriage was failing, I knew I needed a career to provide for my family. I also knew that I wanted to ultimately have a career in the health care industry and that meant returning to college. I obtained student loans, found after-school care for my children and became a nontraditional student at Texas Tech University. I spent two years taking the leveling courses necessary to get into medical school. Honestly, these were some of the most difficult years of my life because of the physical and mental stamina required.

I finally stepped back enough to evaluate the situation and determine that I needed to do something, still in health care, but involving less time. Dietetics was a perfect fit for me because I had a passion for nutrition and the role it plays in our health. It still required two more years of schooling and an internship to end up with my master's in nutrition to become a registered dietitian. During those years, I survived on little sleep and less money. Loving and caring for four elementary-age children is wonderful, but exhausting. In addition, following my dream was requiring a great deal of time and energy from me. Needless to say, I was spread too thin. Then, just as I was thinking I couldn't take any more, more paid a visit.

In the summer of 1994, I found myself at rock bottom. It seemed as though everything that could go wrong—did. After years of counseling, my marriage ended. I suddenly found myself the struggling single mom of four kids. I was in the final semester of my graduate degree. My father was battling the final stages of advanced prostate cancer. My oldest daughter was diagnosed with an eating disorder and placed in an inpatient facility 400 miles away, and my ex-husband took me to court to battle for custody of our children. I was exhausted. I felt pulled in a million directions. I knew I wasn't properly handling my responsibilities as a student, a daughter or a mom. I felt guilty for all I had tried to tackle, and I felt angry (mostly at God) that so many hurdles had been placed in my path in spite of my efforts to be perfect. During my early married years, I had spent an incredible amount of energy creating the image of a perfect family. We started a family right away and I had the responsibility of raising four children by the time I was 27. I took my responsibility seriously and worked hard to be the best mom I could be. It was important to me to be active and involved, so I taught Bible studies, led prayer groups, volunteered, did aerobics, hosted a cooking club ... and worked hard to create the image to appear as though I had it all together. Now, my perfect world was crashing down around me and I was too exhausted—physically and mentally—to know how to move forward.

I wish I could tell you that I just woke up one morning and everything was better, but that is not how it happened.

The next few months were a dull blur—you know, just kind of going through the motions, but feeling totally shut off from emotion or feeling. Reality was too painful, so I just did what I could to make it through the day. Slowly, a change of seasons took place in my life. I finished my internship and obtained my first job as a registered dietitian. My father passed away. My daughter had a breakthrough in her therapy and was eventually able to come back home. I got custody of my children. The healings were slow. The scars were deep. We made it through. Today, my children actually enjoy getting together to recount the horror stories of growing up in a hectic, single-parent home. I think it must be like getting together with your military unit and recalling foxhole stories.

We survived, so the stories now are funny—but at the time, not so much.

One of the most important things I did during this time was to allow myself to evolve. Part of getting your second wind is learning to release your grip on all the extras you are trying to bring along with you and just focus on staying the course. I had no energy left to continue the façade. My imperfect life was laid bare for all to see. I had no choice but to become real, no more performing, no more pretending. Finally, I was able to be me—not who I thought others in my life wanted or expected me to be.

Often when you get caught up in trying to please others, you give little thought to what pleases you. Rediscovering yourself can be tricky because you have no idea where to start. With little sense of direction, and even less energy to reinvent yourself, it is easy to find yourself lost in a haze.

In my search for identity, I was looking for something—anything—to give me purpose and direction. I needed uninterrupted "me" time to heal. I desperately needed to get my second wind. I found it through running.

Turns out I am a runner, although I didn't discover it until I was about 40 years old. I started by running a block, then walking a block for 30 minutes each day. I was soon running more than I was walking, but I couldn't imagine how people could run several miles at a time without taking walk breaks. I did notice, however, that I was beginning to feel better about myself—inside and out. That feeling kept me running.

Call it endorphins. Call it the wind in your face. Soon I was hooked. I entered a five-kilometer race. I ran part and walked part, but I finished. I kept training and ran even longer races. I connected with a coach who gave me a training plan. I joined a running group. I got faster and my fitness level increased. Now it was official. By uncovering my inner athlete, I found a healthy way to escape the quagmire my life had become.

I love running and what it represents in my life. It became my passion—something I could pour myself into. I could do it for me. It gave me time alone with my thoughts. It gave me the courage and the confidence I needed to change my life.

I would be remiss if I didn't share the other thing running did for me. It gave me time alone with God. He and I have had lots of great talks during my runs. I was angry at Him for all the bad things that had happened to mess up my perfect life, so we had lots of heated discussions. I assumed He was disappointed that I hadn't been able to keep up my "Christian façade." Amazingly, I found He loves me just the way I am. Running improved my confidence, but the strength and courage I needed to pick up the pieces and start again came from renewing my relationship with Jesus Christ. True to God's promise, as I've learned to rely more on Him and not my own perfection, He has been faithful to gently mold and shape my rough edges into the person he wants me to be.

Taking charge of your life is all about enduring hardships, overcoming obstacles and having dogged determination to pursue your dreams. It is embracing your sense of adventure to try new things. I've shared with you how in the midst of intense personal struggle, I began to find my second wind. Now it's time to turn the focus to you. If you are searching for how to get started down your own path to wellness, these ideas might help you begin.

Step 1: Take Charge of Your Destiny:

God has a plan for your life—it is up to you to find and follow it. Consider these tips for clearing the clutter in your life so you can discover God's plan for you:

1. **Open Your Eyes to Life's Simple Pleasures.**
Remember as a kid when you entered into experiences with all your heart? You felt the full flood of emotions. Think about the first time you were pushed on a swing. Remember the exhilaration of flying through the air—the wind blowing through your hair, the feeling of flying up and back, then learning to pump yourself higher and higher with your legs? This is the way all of life is meant to be lived—trying new things, experiencing new activities, meeting new people. Be willing to be a kid again. Just as I did with running, begin to identify what new interest you could develop that would give you the energy to begin taking charge of your life.

2. **Open Your Heart to Find Your Passion.**
What moves you? What motivates you to grow and stretch? What people and organizations could benefit from your energy and compassion? Giving your time and energy for the benefit of others is one of the best ways to find adventure and create a winning, rewarding life. I knew I had the desire and the ability to care for patients—to help give them hope and lead them toward health. It was and is my one of my greatest passions. I came to realize that to live my passion; I had to go back to school. What will following your passion require of you?

3. **Choose to Get in the Game.**
To play to win, you can't settle for watching from the sidelines. Most of us have been conditioned to resist change and fear failure. Much like the lion in the *Wizard of Oz*, the first step may be to discover your courage. With that newfound courage, it is time to take your leap of faith into this game of life. Find an activity that allows you to follow your passion, stretch out of your comfort zone and do it. This is the most difficult step. It requires action and com-

mitment from you. What do you need to do to get in the game?

4. Stretch yourself.

During my job as a corporate dietitian at United Super-markets in Lubbock, Texas, I had the opportunity to train dietetic intern students to work in nontraditional dietetic roles. I had an unusual job for a dietitian, and it was a great chance to stretch their minds and their expectations of the jobs they could pursue with a nutrition degree. I did a lot of work in television and radio and made numerous public-speaking appearances. I helped United develop an organic and natural food section and create an original line of ready-to-eat foods. These responsibilities were not things I had been officially trained for in my graduate program, but I had the basic skills and knowledge to do the task—I just needed the courage to pull it off. I had a favorite saying I used with students. It has served me well in my life, and I believe it is the key to learning to be adventurous:

When asked to do a task that stretches you beyond your comfort zone, just say a resounding "yes" and scramble like crazy behind the scenes to make it happen.

What are you doing to actively pursue your dream? Is it requiring more of you than you ever thought you were capable of doing? If not, stretch. You must stretch to grow.

5. Never give up.

You will experience some amazing new adventures as you begin to stretch yourself. Recognize some will be successes and some will be failures. Understand sometimes you must persevere. I recently did a phone interview on national radio, and I didn't think it went all that well for a variety of reasons. But, after I beat myself up for a couple of minutes, I said, "I know I want to do more of these, so what can I do to make sure it goes better next time?" And then I made a list of what I learned from my less-than-stellar performance. I could have said, "I'm not good at radio interviews; I'll never do that again." That would have been giving up. Instead I learned from my mistakes, and I'll nail it next time.

Have you gotten far enough out of your comfort zone to fail? If not, it is time to get out there and take a risk. What is the next step you need to take that feels like a step into completely unknown and uncomfortable territory for you? Take it.

Discovering the courage to get your second wind will give your life incredible meaning and purpose. It will fill your days with joy and excitement as you stretch and grow into all you can possibly be. Dig deep into your soul and allow the real you to emerge. Take time to rediscover your sense of adventure. Use it to pursue your dreams and passions. If you do this, your life will become more rewarding than you ever dreamed possible.

Chapter 2

Be Courageous

"Far better it is to dare mighty things, to win glorious triumphs, even though checkered by failure, than to take rank with those poor spirits who neither enjoy much nor suffer much, because they live in the grey twilight that knows not victory nor defeat."
—THEODORE ROOSEVELT

"Life shrinks or expands in proportion to one's courage."
—ANAIS NIN

"Two roads diverged in a wood, and I—I took the one less traveled by, and that has made all the difference."
—ROBERT FROST

I am convinced taking charge of your destiny by adopting a healthier way of life requires more courage than most are willing to muster. As we go through life, it is much easier and more comfortable to conform to behaviors we see modeled around us than it is to stand up for what is best. The quotes you have just read are some of my favorites when it comes to living a life of courage. Here is one of my own:

"Courage is discovered by stretching out of your comfort zone and stepping into the unknown—knowing that whatever happens could change your life forever."

As we explore what it takes to build a healthy body, it will become clear that deciding to take charge of your body requires great courage. Too many people today practice an if-it-feels-good-do-it lifestyle. In our fast-paced lives, whatever is easy is replacing discipline and self-control. Little time seems to exist for cooking and gathering the family around the dinner table for a healthy meal. Because of that, a majority choose to rush to the fast-food drive-through and grab anything quick and filling. As for exercise, most people would rather sleep another hour than roll out of bed to work out. Deciding to follow the healthy road less traveled in life requires courage—the courage to take a stand, swim against the current and change behavior.

If you have made poor eating and fitness choices, you may be looking in the mirror at a body that seems hopeless to change. I want to encourage you by reminding you that you created your body by making a series of poor choices, and you will create a new, healthier body just the same way—one small, courageous step at a time. These small victories build confidence. As confidence in our ability to make small changes increases, the courage to make big changes will follow.

To give you a good mental picture of this kind of courage, let me share a story. It takes place in Panama—a beautiful country with lush rain forests and many picturesque rivers and lakes. My parents lived blocks from Gatun Lake, where we spent many happy summer days when we visited. Early during their time in Panama, my brother and his wife visited. We have a great video of my newly married brother, Lal, and his wife, Terri, standing on a two-story dock overlooking Gatun Lake. In the video, he is trying to encourage her to jump off the dock into the lake below.

Encourage really is too mild a word. He had already jumped many times and knew how fun it was. He wanted her to experience it. She walked to the edge, ready to take the plunge, but lost her courage at the last minute and walked back. He talked sweetly to her, telling her how wonderful it would be and how much she would love it. She walked to the edge once again, started to jump but then turned at the last minute and ran back to safety. This went on for what seemed like forever. She wanted to jump. She began walking toward the edge, then got scared and ran back to where she felt safe.

Aren't we the same way when trying to find the courage we need to make a big change in our lives? We want to change. We know it would be rewarding, but it would mean taking a leap of faith into unknown territory. We keep getting close to the edge, really toying with the idea of changing, but few of us ever muster the courage to take the plunge. By the way, after several false alarms, Terri did finally jump off the dock and she and Lal spent a delightful day jumping off the dock and swimming in the lake. The moral: Regardless of how long it takes you to find your courage, it is never too late to take the leap.

Overcoming fear is one of the most important things you can do to lay the groundwork for success in adopting a healthy lifestyle. Fear often is what keeps you running in place. It thwarts individual potential and prevents you from becoming all you can be. When you are fearful, the focus is on all that could possibly go wrong rather than envisioning the rewards that will come with success. Courageous people are not without fears; they just take the plunge and act despite their fears.

We all know people who demonstrate great courage. If you've never been described as courageous, it is not too late. You can take action and develop the courage needed to become the person you want to be.

I witnessed a powerfully courageous act begin to unfold in 1999 at a Team in Training meeting in my home. I was working for United Supermarkets at that time, and I was serving on the board of the local diabetes council. I had heard about their national Team in Training program. I invited several fellow runners to view a video and explore the idea of training and raising money for diabetes by running a marathon in Kona, Hawaii.

I announced the meeting at my office to solicit runners. As the group was gathering, I answered the door to find Claudette, a woman from my office who had just been diagnosed with diabetes. I had worked to help her understand how to treat her condition with diet and exercise. I had encouraged her to lose weight to gain better control over her diabetes. Claudette is one of the sweetest people I know, but she is shy and withdrawn. It must have been extremely difficult for her to find the courage to show up at my home for the meeting.

We started talking about who would be interested in training for Kona. Claudette spoke up and said, "I know I cannot run a marathon, but I want to train with you guys. I will make the commitment to walk all the miles that you run. I need to do this for myself and for all those with diabetes." I wasn't sure she was fully aware of the commitment she was making, but I was proud of her willingness to step out of her comfort zone. We found a coach and began an eight-month training program. True to her commitment, Claudette was with us. If we ran five miles, she walked five miles. If we did 10, she did 10.

She started before us and left long after we finished. By the time we left for Kona, she had lost more than 80 pounds. She had gained such control over her diabetes that her doctor took her off her oral medication. Her self-confidence was amazing to watch. I roomed with her in Kona, and I wish I could completely describe the intense personal stretch and growth the experience provided for her. First of all, she had never flown, she had never been out of Texas, she had never seen the ocean, and she had never been in a race. We stayed in a great hotel and were a part of a throng of people in Hawaii racing to fight diabetes. She was moved by the experience. The night before the race, she was scared and intently focused on working through her fears, but absolutely determined to follow through with her dream of finishing. The next day at the race, she walked like a champion. I've never been more proud. She faced her fears, conquered them, and finished strong.

If Claudette can find the courage, regardless of the cost, you can, too. So here you are standing poised and ready to make the leap toward healthy living. You've mentally prepared for the challenges that lie ahead; now it's time to take the first step. Getting started takes more courage than anything else you'll do to get to your goal. The time has come for you to conquer your fear and start your joyful journey toward health and wellness.

Deciding to abandon the status quo to begin making healthy lifestyle choices is not easy. You will confront obstacles and hurdles along the way. Here are some suggestions for turning potential pitfalls into stepping stones to success:

Pitfall: Weak support system.
Plan for success: Build pockets of strength.

I try to identify a person's support system whenever I am working with new clients. I am interested in knowing what they have in place to help them reach their goals. This can make all the difference because few can make such a major change alone.

Have you noticed the one thing almost all obese people have at home? Often when I ask that question in presentations to other health care professionals, typical answers are a television or a comfortable recliner. The correct answer, though, is this: other obese people.

Being overweight and living a lifestyle that leads to obesity is something generally learned from parents and passed on to children. I once hosted a booth at a wellness fair for a large corporation. About 5,000 people attended, and my staff and I were astounded by the number of obese families that passed our booth. The children were like miniature clones of their overweight parents. This illustrates why it takes courage to make these decisions. It is more than proclaiming your choice to live healthy. You will battle family norms those around you still participate in, meaning they may be unintentionally less supportive of your decision to change.

I know you are familiar with the saying, "Misery loves company." Even if those who love you pledge to support your decision, they may unwittingly do little things to undermine your success. It is not as much fun to stop for a triple scoop of ice cream if the person you are with is not indulging. Instead of encouraging you in your bold decision not to consume such a decadent treat, they might tell you, "Oh, it won't matter just this once," or "You're no fun anymore." It takes an enormous amount of courage and determination to stay the course and stand your ground.

To overcome this stumbling block, you need to identify and develop pockets of support from people who will encourage and affirm your efforts. I've found these ideas to be helpful in combating a weak support system:

- Find a friend or family member who has similar weight loss and fitness goals. It is even better if they are someone you work with, live close to, or live with, so you can eat meals together and work out together.

- If you can't find a weight-loss buddy, look for a group at your office, your church or community center who share you goals. Who knows? This could be a great chance to meet some new friends who are committed to healthier living, just like you.

- Go to a local running store, YMCA, or community center to see if they have walking groups, cycling groups or running groups you can join. Committing to a group fitness activity is a great way to find a small pocket of support for your new way of life.

Pitfall: No time.
Plan for success: Take time.

Despite all we hear about not having time, one thing remains true: We all have the same amount of time every day. The key to carving out time to get healthy is to be ruthless— cut out the fluff and replace it with purposeful behavior.

Some of the busiest people I know also are the healthiest. They find a workout time that works for them, and then they sacredly guard that time against any conflicting scheduling. Whether it is at 5 a.m., noon, after work or late evening, that time is non-negotiable.

I have a friend who is in senior management for a global food company. He lives in Minnesota, where brutally cold temperatures often can be a challenge. For as long as I've known him, he gets up at 4:30 a.m. to run. A handful of days during the winter months force him to the gym to use the treadmill, but the other 350-plus days each year, he and three buddies meet in the dark for a four-mile run before work.

That's commitment. That's taking time to stay fit. Knowing he is running in the cold and snow of Minnesota often is a great motivator for me. I tell myself, "If he can do it there, surely I have no excuse to avoid running in South Texas."

Pitfall: Healthy foods taste like cardboard.
Plan for success: Learn to fill your plate with flavor and color.

Once you begin replacing high-fat, high-flavor foods with healthy foods, you might miss the intense flavors and creamy textures in your mouth. This common pitfall confronts anyone beginning a healthy eating plan. The good news is studies indicate it takes only about one month to retrain your taste buds to enjoy a healthier way of eating. If you will commit to a diet of fresh fruits and vegetables, green leafy salads, whole grains and lean meats, you will be amazed at how your body begins to crave those foods. Your energy level will increase. Your blood pressure may begin to normalize. Your weight will begin to drop. No longer will it be a sacrifice to eat that way. Instead, it will be a pleasure to fuel your body with healthy foods.

You don't have to add fat to add flavor and color to your diet. You can intensify flavor by adding veggies such as mushrooms, peppers, onions and tomatoes to your favorite recipes. You can enhance the flavor of savory recipes in a number of ways:

- Try apples, apricots, peaches or mangoes with pork or chicken recipes.

- Pair raspberries or cherries with beef recipes.

- Create a fresh fruit salsa spiced with fruit and peppers to use as a topping for grilled fish, chicken or pork.

- Provide a burst of flavor for fish with lemon or lime juice.

- Learn to use fresh herbs to season foods without adding sodium or calories.

Explore the possibilities of increasing flavor and color. You will find healthy eating can be an exciting new adventure instead of a pitfall to be avoided.

Pitfall: I hate to work out.
Plan for success: Find activities you enjoy and learn to excel.

Increasing your activity level is a challenge. Many people do not enjoy going to the gym and sweating. If that is you, try a different approach. Find a sport or activity you've always wanted to participate in, and then become proficient at it by taking lessons and committing yourself to a dedicated practice schedule.

I played in a tennis league one spring. One of the ladies in my league was undoubtedly a tennis novice. One night after practice, I started talking to her. Her story made such an impression on me. It turns out her husband had recently died, and she felt miserable and alone. She was spending her days eating in front of the television. Her weight was ballooning, and her energy was sagging. She had a talk with herself and decided that hiding away was not a solution. She wanted to find something fun to fill her time, so she decided to get active by doing something she always wanted to do—play tennis.

She took lessons, signed up for a league and began playing several times a week. She said it saved her life. Before tennis, she was lonely and depressed about not being able to grow old with the love of her life. By pouring herself into learning to play tennis, she discovered new energy, a new set of friends who shared her love for tennis, and a new fitness tool that seemed more like fun than work.

Pitfall: My mom made me clean my plate, and I don't know how to stop until all my food is gone and I'm stuffed.
Plan for success: Get in touch with your hunger. Eat when you are hungry and stop when you are full.

I bet most of us heard the clean-your-plate message while growing up. We hate to be wasteful. As we are throwing out leftovers, we mentally remind ourselves of "those starving children in China" who would dearly love to have food to eat. Mind you, I'm not advocating waste, but solutions can be found to avoid overeating, even when cleaning your plate. Fill your plate with the correct portion. Then, even when you clean your plate, you will not be overstuffed. If you like the look of a full plate of food, try eating on smaller plates. Your smaller portion will visually appear larger.

A number of studies have been done recently regarding people's ability to get in touch with their hunger. The graph below is an excellent tool to help visualize your true hunger. You want to stop eating when you are at neutral or satisfied.

Remember, it takes your brain 20 minutes to catch up with your stomach, so the trick is to stop before you are above 5 on the scale.

Identify and Honor Your True Hunger

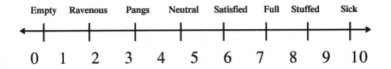

Take the 'Apple Test'!

A good measuring stick is the apple test. When you are eating and feel yourself getting satisfied, before reaching for more food, ask, "Would I eat an apple right now?" If the answer is yes, then you might still be hungry and need a little more food. However, if the answer is no, then you are over-eating and need to push away from the table.

> **Pitfall:** I'm always looking for the quick fix of a fad diet.
> **Plan for success:** If something sounds too good to be true—it usually is. Don't fall victim to the fad-diet cycle. Spend your energy getting healthy and let the weight loss take care of itself.

I always remind my clients that it took a long time to get into their predicament, and it is going to take some time to get out. No quick answer to losing a significant amount of weight can be found. Whether you are more than 100 pounds overweight or 10 pounds overweight, you need to aim for a 1½- to 2-pound weight loss each week.

Do the math—if you need to lose 100 pounds, it will probably take you about a year. The key to success is getting off the diet rollercoaster and investing time in getting healthy. The diagram below indicates how fad dieting can become a vicious cycle. If you start an extreme diet asking you to consume fewer than 1,200 calories per day, it will not take long to get too hungry to continue. Then, before you know it, deprivation will get the best of you. The diet goes by the wayside, and you begin eating everything in sight. Next comes the feeling of failure, the resulting weight gain, and the guilt associated with not ever being able to be a successful dieter. Soon you give in to the guilt and start the process again.

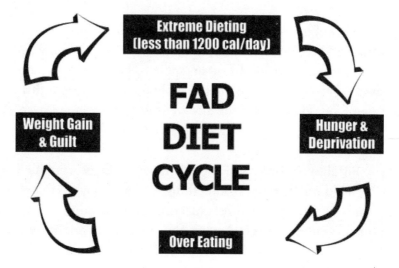

The best way to avoid this vicious cycle is not to be suckered into quick-fix weight-loss schemes. Instead, determine to be patient and commit to an active lifestyle built around a nutrient-rich diet of fresh fruits and vegetables, whole grains, low-fat dairy and lean meats.

In this chapter, we've explored what it takes to develop the courage to get started down the path to health and well-being. We have identified the pitfalls that might detour your success and made a plan for overcoming them. We know courage is available to everyone who would *choose* to conquer their fears.

In the words of Winston Churchill,

"Destiny is not a matter of chance, it is a matter of ***choice****; it is not a thing to be waited for, it is a thing to be achieved."*

So, here you are, poised and ready to make the leap toward healthy living. You have mentally prepared for the challenges ahead. Now it is time to take the first step.

It is time to take the plunge.

CHAPTER 3

Fuel to Succeed:
Seek Balance

*For you formed my inward parts; you knitted me
together in my mother's womb. I praise you, for I am
fearfully and wonderfully made. Wonderful are your
works; my soul knows it very well.*

PSALM 139:13-14

Our bodies are amazing. Stop and think about how the parts of your body work together to keep you healthy and strong. It is truly a miracle.

The key to creating a healthy body is finding and maintaining that delicate balance between the foods you consume and the activities you enjoy.

God designed an amazing plan for how our bodies will function. Amazingly, He also gave us the choice of how to care for our bodies. For instance, if we choose to gorge ourselves on junk food and neglect getting enough exercise, our bodies will likely respond by gaining an exorbitant amount of weight. The result of adopting this lifestyle is a sluggish body highly prone to behavioral diseases such as obesity, type 2 diabetes, heart disease, and some types of cancer. On the other extreme, if we decide to underfeed our bodies, we will become frail and will likely develop conditions such as anorexia and bulimia. Either extreme of disordered eating is generally catastrophic.

I experienced firsthand the pain of disordered eating with my oldest daughter, Leigh. I am recounting the story now with her permission. Because her story has a happy ending, she is willing and able to offer help and hope to many young women and their families as they struggle to manage this awful disease that plagues so many in our society.

Leigh's story begins like this:

I took my two younger children to Panama to visit my parents. My husband and the two older girls were planning to join us two weeks later for an extended family vacation. When they got off the plane, I couldn't believe how thin and gaunt Leigh looked. I was concerned but tried to brush it off as a passing phase. She was 12, and little did I know at the time, this was the beginning of what was to become a long, arduous ordeal. Leigh was eating next to nothing, and we could not beg or force her to eat.

We even went to the Pizza Hut on the military base in Panama, thinking surely she would eat pizza. All she ate was a piece of lettuce and a crust off her sister's pizza, so I knew we were in trouble. For the next several years, she and our family were in and out of counseling. We had times when we thought she was getting better because she was eating, but we soon sadly discovered she was just tired of fighting the hunger and made the decision to switch from anorexia to bulimia. Both diseases are horrible examples of the trauma that disordered eating can wreak on the body.

We watched in horror as Leigh went from a vibrant, beautiful, gifted student and athlete to a frail 90 pounds of skin and bones. This went on for several years. Shortly after her 16th birthday, she and her boyfriend had been swimming and then went for a snowcone, when Leigh passed out in the parking lot. He took her to the hospital and called me. I met them there, and the physician caring for her said she was very ill and refused to release her except to an inpatient facility.

We took her to a treatment center in San Antonio where she stayed three months. It was a tough experience for her, but she finally had a breakthrough and was able to return home. The healing process for eating disorders is similar to other addictive behaviors—it is something she will deal with the rest of her life. It causes all kinds of lasting body trauma—such as heart problems, a decrease in bone density, and a variety of hormonal issues. Through the grace of God, she is strong and healthy and back to her athletic self. She is a professional runner and track coach at a Midwest university and has been well now for almost 10 years. It is such a blessing to see her pursuing her dreams and enjoying life again.

Thankfully, our bodies are wonderfully made. They are resilient and able to handle a lot of abuse. Regardless of how we feed and care for them, they seem to work overtime to try to keep us healthy and balanced—at least during our youth. However, as we age, this begins to catch up with us. If we have been mostly sedentary and thrived on junk food, our body systems have had to work in overdrive to try to keep us healthy. This puts major strain on our bodies and can result in many of the behavioral diseases we see showing up in midlife.

Learning to eat healthy is not a diet; it is a lifestyle change.

Make no mistake, this is not a diet book. It is about how to get and stay healthy—for life. Changing the way you fuel your body can be the most important step. Toward that end, this chapter will focus on healthy eating as we create a plan that includes a balanced variety of the nutrients required to build and maintain a healthy body.

Misinformation on healthy eating is virtually everywhere in the media today. It seems whenever you turn on the television or pick up a newspaper, someone is hyping a new weight-loss gimmick or the latest information on a new food shown to be the secret to the fountain of youth. And, even mainstream news reports seem to highlight a "food de jour" that can help protect against cancer or heart disease. It is no wonder the general public is frustrated, confused, and often unsure of whom to trust for sound nutritional advice.

Keep two important things in mind when evaluating nutritional information. First, if it sounds too good to be true, it probably is. Make sure to evaluate the research and verify that the findings have been substantiated in peer-reviewed journals. Second, if the findings are extreme, encouraging you to eliminate a nutrient group completely (for example: no carbohydrates) or if the diet is focusing too much attention on one particular food (for example: grapefruit), steer clear.

As you read this book, trust that I endorse only validated research and rely on professional sources that practice credible science. As a registered dietitian with years of experience in helping people take control of their health, I can reduce my key nutrition message to one sentence:

The foods you consume and the physical activities you enjoy will determine your physical and mental health as you age.

It is time to get back to nutrition basics. As you begin to take control of how you feed your body, you will want to focus your attention of understanding the basic building blocks of a healthy diet. Once you do, your path to a healthy lifestyle will become much clearer.

1. A healthy body is built on real food.

If you are making wise choices in the foods you select, you will be able to receive all the nutrients your body needs to be healthy and strong. To confidently select good-for-you foods, let me refresh your memory on some nutrition basics:

Nutrition truth: Your body needs carbohydrates, protein, and healthy fat to function at its best.

- **Carbohydrates** are your body's first choice for energy, providing readily accessible fuel for physical performance. Carbohydrates are "brain food"; they are the nutrient your brain prefers to use for fuel. They also provide dietary fiber that helps keep the digestive system functioning correctly.

- **Protein** is used by your body to build and repair body tissues and muscle. Proteins provide building blocks of the enzymes and hormones that keep our bodies in good working order.

- **Fat** is important for slowing the digestive process so you are not hungry an hour after eating a meal. It adds flavor and a creamy texture to the foods we eat. It also aids in the absorption of fat-soluble vitamins, which include vitamins A, D, E, and K.

Each of these major nutrient categories plays a unique role in nourishing your body, and a healthy diet must contain a good balance of all three. A healthy diet is built on the 40-30-30 rule—40 percent of calories from carbohydrates, 30 percent from protein and 30 percent from fat.

2. **When adopting a healthy diet, it is important to remember not all carbohydrates, proteins and fats are created equal.**

> **Nutrition truth:** To get the biggest nutritional bang for your buck, be sure to choose a variety of foods within each nutrient category.

A brief primer on how to make the best choices within each nutrient category:

- **Carbohydrate:** Be sure you choose complex carbohydrates that are broken down into glucose more slowly than simple carbohydrates and thus provide a steady stream of energy throughout the day. Good choices for complex carbohydrates include whole grain breads, cereals, pasta, brown rice, corn, beans, and potatoes. The simple carbohydrates you select need to come from fruits and vegetables. Each provides its own package of vitamins and minerals the body needs to function at its best.

- **Protein:** Choose lean protein to get the benefit without adding all the saturated fat that comes along with higher fat animal protein sources. Beans and nuts are also great sources.

- **Fat:** To select the calories in your diet from fat, choose unsaturated fats such as avocados, nuts, olive oil, canola oil, and fatty fish like salmon.

3. **All foods can fit into a healthy diet.**

   Nutrition truth: If you learn to balance your intake with the calories you expend, all the foods you love can fit into your healthy eating plan.

The key is working each day to balance the amount of fuel you take in with the amount of energy you expend. My background is in culinary and I enjoy nothing more than delicious foods that awaken my taste buds with complexity of flavor and texture. My friends and family will tell you—I enjoy a wide variety of foods, I eat reasonable portions, and I do a lot of running to help counteract my love for good food. If I had to completely give up butter, cream, and a good steak, I'm not sure life would be worth living.

4. **We must retrain ourselves to eat at regularly scheduled intervals throughout the day.**

   Nutrition truth: A regulated eating plan provides an important physiological function. It keeps blood sugar stable and metabolism revved up throughout the day.

The ideal eating plan is based on three meals and three snacks eaten at about the same time each day. An average-sized 40 year old woman needs about 1800 calories a day to maintain a healthy weight. In this case, a good plan would be to keep the three meals approximately equivalent in calories

(~450 calories each) and the snacks equivalent (~150 calories each). This allows your body to rely on the fact that you will feed it every 2 to 3 hours. In turn, it responds by burning the calories you consume in a most efficient manner, rather than hanging on to every calorie you consume in fear that you may not feed it again for an extended period of time.

5. The foods you eat can boost your energy or sap your energy.

It is 4 p.m. and you're dragging. You are in dire need of an energy boost to make it through the rest of the afternoon. What do you grab? Well, too often, the answer is a candy bar and a soft drink. If you've ever done this, you know the energy boost is great for about 30 minutes, but soon you feel even worse than you did before the high-calorie, high-sugar fix you gave yourself. Why? The simple carbohydrates are quickly absorbed into your blood stream, giving your body a quick shot of energy. When that energy is metabolized, your blood sugar drops quickly, leaving you with no energy and feeling awful. Consider the same 4 p.m. scenario, but this time grab six or eight almonds and a few dried apricots. The combination of healthy fat, protein and carbohydrate will help satisfy your hunger and give you the energy you need to last until dinner.

> **Nutrition truth:** A good mix of protein, healthy fats, and carbohydrates takes longer to digest and leaves you feeling energized until your next meal.

This is a list of behaviors that can either boost or drain your energy. Choose more energy gainers to be successful in building your eating plan.

Energy Drainers vs. Energy Gainers

Skipping breakfast	Fueling up with a balanced breakfast that includes protein
Eating too many or too few carbs	Balancing your intake at each meal with a mix of carbs, proteins and fats
Living on junk food	Building your diet on nutrient-rich foods
Eating too much, too often	Consuming properly sized portions
Not eating enough	Honoring your true hunger
Being a "couch potato"	Getting and staying fit

6. **Nutrient-rich foods should build the core of our daily dietary intake.**

Recently, I was doing some consulting work for a large corporation. The gentleman I was working with on the account was a committed cyclist and an overcommitted businessman. Between the hours he worked and the hours he trained, he had little time to shop or plan meals. He sought my advice on the foods he could use to build a healthy eating plan to enhance his performance.

> **Nutrition truth:** Whether you are fueling for performance or just eating to maximize your energy to meet the demands of your day, nutrient-packed superfoods can play a key role in getting and keeping you healthy.

I recommend this list of 10 superfoods to my clients and include brief descriptions of why they are important. These are not the only foods that will provide the nutrition you need to build a healthy body, but for those of you who want a suggested shopping list, here you go:

- **Almonds:** Munch on this heart-healthy snack to give you a nutritious boost and keep you satisfied between meals. Good source of manganese, copper, and Vitamin B2 (Riboflavin)—all of which play a key role in energy production. Promotes colon health—one-quarter cup equals four grams of fiber. Excellent source of vitamin E and monounsaturated fat shown to reduce LDL cholesterol levels and decrease risk of heart disease.

- **Avocados:** Bright green, lusciously creamy and full of healthy monounsaturated fats important in lowering LDL cholesterol and promoting heart health. This fat in avocados also helps increase the absorption of carotenoids in vegetables such as carrots, lettuce and spinach.

- **Beans:** Red and yellow, black and white … and everything in between, legumes are extremely versatile to use in appetizers, salads, and entrees. They are a great source of soluble fiber, which is helpful in glucose management and reducing LDL cholesterol. They are an excellent source of protein and high in antioxidants. The darker the color of the bean, the higher the antioxidant level.

- **Blueberries:** Researchers at Tufts University analyzed 60 fruits and vegetables for their antioxidant capability. Blueberries ranked first in their capacity to destroy free radicals. Research also shows blueberries may just be the best food on the planet to preserve a young brain as we mature—their powerful antioxidant activity protects our brain from oxidative stress.

- **Low-fat dairy:** An easy, tasty way to protect your teeth and bones. It provides a low-cost, high-quality source of protein. It is a good source of vitamin D and calcium—two nutrients essential to bone health, and vitamin A, which is important for strong immune function.

- **Oats:** These provide anti-cancer activity equal to or higher than that of fruits and vegetables. They lower bad cholesterol levels and provide unique antioxidants proven to decrease the risk of cardiovascular disease.

- **Salmon:** This is a superfood for your heart, joints, and memory. Reel some in two or three times a week. Salmon is low in calories and saturated fat, yet high in protein, and omega-3 essential fatty acids important in promoting heart health.

- **Spinach:** Powerful anti-inflammatory properties protect against arthritis and antioxidants to protect against cancer and heart disease. It is an excellent source of vitamins A, C, and K, and is a good source of folate and magnesium, providing protection from cardiovascular disease.

- **Sweet potatoes:** This nutritional all-star keeps your skin young and helps prevent damage from sunlight. Sweet potatoes contain high levels of vitamins A and C, which are powerful antioxidants working in the body to eliminate free radicals.

- **Tomatoes:** They are high in vitamins A and C, dietary fiber, and lycopene. Eating these may help decrease the risk of prostate cancer as well as breast, lung and stomach cancers.

7. Eat when you are hungry and stop when you are full.

This sounds like obvious advice, but it seems we've totally learned to ignore our hunger cues.

> **Nutrition truth:** Learning to pay attention to your body, feeding it when you're hungry and pushing away from the table when you are full is the most valuable weight-loss tool you'll ever find.

We eat for many reasons other than physical hunger. Think about the times you eat when not hungry. Is it from boredom? Loneliness? Stress? Pleasure? Reward? When we eat for reasons other than physical hunger, we often reach for comfort foods—high-fat, high-calorie splurges that may leave us feeling even less satisfied than when we started our mindless eating binge.

8. Develop an eating plan based on healthy foods you enjoy.

> **Nutrition truth:** When you make the decision to adopt a healthy lifestyle, you will be more successful if you build a plan that is not overly restrictive and includes many foods you love.

Before you build your personal eating plan, you'll need to do some calculations. Be sure you know your Body Mass Index (BMI) and the calorie level you need each day to maintain your weight. If you need to lose weight, I recommend a 25 percent calorie deficit to produce a 1 ½- to 2-pound weight loss each week.

Body Mass Index (BMI):

BMI is a statistical measure of your weight scaled according to your height. It equals a person's weight in kilograms divided by height in meters squared. BMI is an objective measurement tool often used by health professionals to discuss matters related to being overweight or underweight more objectively with their patients.

Risk of Associated Disease According to BMI and Waist Size

BMI		Waist less than or equal to 40 in. (men) or 35 in. (women)	Waist greater than 40 in. (men) or 35 in. (women)
18.5 or less	Underweight	--	N/A
18.5–24.9	Normal	--	N/A
25.0–29.9	Overweight	Increased	High
30.0–34.9	Obese	High	Very High
35.0–39.9	Obese	Very High	Very High
40 or greater	Extremely Obese	Extremely High	Extremely High

Determining Your Body Mass Index (BMI)

The table below has already done the math and metric conversions. To use the table, find the appropriate height in the left-hand column. Move across the row to the given weight. The number at the top of the column is the BMI for that height and weight.

BMI (kg/m²)	19	20	21	22	23	24	25	26	27	28	29	30	35	40
Height (in.)	Weight (lb.)													
58	91	96	100	105	110	115	119	124	129	134	138	143	167	191
59	94	99	104	109	114	119	124	128	133	138	143	148	173	198
60	97	102	107	112	118	123	128	133	138	143	148	153	179	204
61	100	106	111	116	122	127	132	137	143	148	153	158	185	211
62	104	109	115	120	126	131	136	142	147	153	158	164	191	218
63	107	113	118	124	130	135	141	146	152	158	163	169	197	225
64	110	116	122	128	134	140	145	151	157	163	169	174	204	232
65	114	120	126	132	138	144	150	156	162	168	174	180	210	240
66	118	124	130	136	142	148	155	161	167	173	179	186	216	247
67	121	127	134	140	146	153	159	166	172	178	185	191	223	255
68	125	131	138	144	151	158	164	171	177	184	190	197	230	262
69	128	135	142	149	155	162	169	176	182	189	196	203	236	270
70	132	139	146	153	160	167	174	181	188	195	202	207	243	278
71	136	143	150	157	165	172	179	186	193	200	208	215	250	286
72	140	147	154	162	169	177	184	191	199	206	213	221	258	294
73	144	151	159	166	174	182	189	197	204	212	219	227	265	302
74	148	155	163	171	179	186	194	202	210	218	225	233	272	311
75	152	160	168	176	184	192	200	208	216	224	232	240	279	319
76	156	164	172	180	189	197	205	213	221	230	238	246	287	328

Body weight in pounds according to height and body mass index.

There are many BMI calculators online. Access them by using the search term Body Mass Index in your search engine and entering your height and weight information.

Now that you've determined your BMI and have a general idea of your weight status in relation to your height, it is time to determine how many calories you need to consume each day to either gain, lose or maintain your healthy weight.

Calorie Needs:

In 2005, the American Dietetic Association published a comparison of various equations used to determine basic calorie needs. The Mifflin-St. Jeor equation I am using here was found to be the most accurate. (Helpful hint: For those who can't remember the conversions to metric: 1 inch = 2.54 cm, 1 kg = 2.2 pounds.)

Men
10 x weight (kg) + 6.25 x height (cm) - 5 x age (y) + 5

Women
10 x weight (kg) + 6.25 x height (cm) - 5 x age (y)—161

Ex) (10 x 59 kg) + (6.25 x 163 cm)—(5 x 50)—161
= 1198 calories/day

This gives you the base calorie calculation needed to maintain your current weight. Our bodies need calories for daily functions such as breathing, digestion, and daily activities. Weight gain occurs when calories consumed exceed this need. Physical activity plays a key role in energy balance because it uses up calories consumed. Your basic calorie needs are estimates of how many calories you would burn if you were to do nothing but rest for 24 hours. They represent the minimum amount of energy required to keep your body functioning, including your heart beating, lungs breathing, and body temperature normal.

Since these basic caloric needs only represent resting energy expenditure, an adjustment must be made to reflect your activity level. This is done by multiplying by an activity factor (McArdle et. al. 1996).

Activity Factor	Category	Definition
1.2	Sedentary	Little or no exercise and desk job
1.375	Lightly Active	Light exercise or sports 1-3 days a week
1.55	Moderately Active	Moderate exercise or sports 3-5 days a week
1.725	Very Active	Hard exercise or sports 6-7 days a week
1.9	Extremely Active	Hard daily exercise or sports and physical job

From the female example above, she needs 1,198 calories a day. If she works out 3 to 5 times a week, then multiply that by a moderately active activity level of 1.55. Her total daily calorie need would be:

For Weight Maintenance:
Ex) 1,198 calories x 1.55 = 1,857 calories per day

For Weight Loss:
Calorie Needs—25% ex) 1,857 calories/day—464 calories = 1,393 calories/day

For Weight Gain:
Calorie Needs + 25% ex) 1,857 calories/day + 464 calories = 2,321 calories/day

Once you've completed your calorie calculation, use the following guide to give you the number of servings of each food group to eat each day based on your body's needs.

Calorie Meal Plan (Daily)	1,200	1,500	1,800	2,000	2,500
Starch	5	7	8	9	11
Fruit	3	3	4	4	6
Milk	2	2	3	3	3
Vegetables	2	2	3	4	5
Meat and Meat Substitutes	4	4	6	6	8
Fat	3	4	4	5	6

This chapter is full of information and is a lot to absorb, but it can be life-changing.

Occasionally I will go to a client's house to teach them in their own kitchen how easy it can be to prepare a healthy meal. On one such evening, I was in the home of a client whose husband is diabetic and does not neccessarily follow a healthy lifestyle. She would love for him to eat better and exercise more to help gain control of his diabetes. While we were eating, I shared a story of a diabetic I had been working with who committed herself to a weight loss and exercise plan that changed her life. Over a year's time, she was able to lose almost 100 pounds, get off all diabetes medications, and basically get her health and her life back.

Her husband looked at me and said, "You don't have a job. You have a higher calling. You really are making a difference in people's lives." I appreciated him reminding me of my purpose. It is always a wonderful feeling when someone notices and appreciates your passion. But it is even more rewarding when you are able to help people identify how to get started down their own personal path to health. If you are reading this thinking, "My life is out of control; I'm hopelessly out of balance," then this book is for you. You have the power and resources within yourself to change your life. I want to encourage you to use the information in this chapter to begin to regain your balance and reclaim your life. What changes are necessary in your life to start down your path to wellness?

CHAPTER 4

Fit to Excel: Be Active

Adopting an active lifestyle requires your complete commitment. You will face numerous challenges every day where you will have a choice to make. Life pressures us from every side and we can find excuses for missing our workout on a regular basis. Each time you are faced with a choice between what is best and what feels good for the moment, it will be up to you to choose wisely. Health is a by-product of a disciplined life. How committed will you be to a consistent fitness regimen? Ask yourself this question:

What am I willing to sacrifice for what I want to become?

Whether you are a busy mom trying to juggle a houseful of kids or a busy CEO juggling workplace demands, the challenge remains, "How do I find time for me?" Carving out time for exercise is not easy. Many just throw up their hands and say, "I'd work out, but I simply can't find the time." However, there are those few willing to make the sacrifices necessary to achieve excellence. Some of these are my clients who get up at 4:30 or 5 a.m. every day to work out and then head off to run major corporations. Some are moms with young kids who wake up in time for an early morning run before their husbands leave for work.

Do you remember the commercial several years ago that showed a teenager who was a great athlete and straight-A student? The camera pans to him as he is running across the goal line to make the game-winning touchdown and then moves to someone in the crowd who says to a friend, "Everything comes so easy to him." Next, the commercial pans to scenes of him up early to practice, after school at his job sweeping the floor at a local restaurant, then at home after work in the evening to study. The point is this: Success doesn't come easy to him; he succeeds because he is willing to put in the time it takes to excel. Vince Lombardi said it best, *"The difference between a successful person and others is not a lack of strength, not a lack of knowledge, but rather a lack of will."*

Do you have the courage to dig deep enough into your soul to find the will to become the best you can be? This is the most important question you can ask yourself as you determine to adopt a healthy lifestyle. You will need determination to make wise food choices, to keep a consistent workout schedule and to focus your mind on the good things in your life. Some people are born into families where this behavior is modeled, and some must work harder to figure it out on their own. Regardless of the way you were raised and the circumstances you have faced, you can develop the will to succeed.

As we work through helping you discover a fitness plan you enjoy, the resulting healthy body looking back at you in the mirror will give you confidence. You will no longer feel guilty for your inaction but rather will be proud of yourself for taking charge of your life and health. Your aim will be to learn to "fall in love with fitness."

I often see people in social settings where everyone is

eating, drinking, and having a great time. Then someone asks the question, "So what do you do?" When I say, "I'm a dietitian," it's like someone threw a wet blanket on the party. Immediately people either start apologizing for how they are eating, or they start defending their right to indulge. As a dietitian, I don't want to take away or judge their right to enjoy themselves. I love parties—to me there is nothing better than eating, drinking, and spending time with friends. When this situation arises, I always say, "No worries, it just looks to me like you are carb loading for a really long run tomorrow."

I don't want people to feel embarrassed or guilty for their behavior, but outside of the party setting, I do want to make sure they understand the correlation between indulging and activity. My theory is this: The reason people feel guilty about overindulging in food and drink is they have a major disconnect when it comes to understanding the relationship between how much you consume and how much you weigh. The variable I see between obese people and healthy weight people is they "get it." For them, the message resonates. *The calories you consume must be balanced with the calories you expend in physical activity.*

I don't live in a bubble, and I do recognize the occasional splurge is manageable and, for most of us, a fact of life. However, if someone chooses indulgent behavior as a *lifestyle*, it could likely result in some of the chronic, behaviorally based diseases we see as we age. Acting U.S. Surgeon General Rear Admiral Kenneth P. Moritsugu, M.D., recently published an article in the *Journal of the American Dietetic Association* that read, "By practicing healthful habits early on, many of the consequences associated with chronic disease can be avoided. Good nutrition and regular physical activity work together to promote health and independence for older adults. Promoting healthful lifestyles of older people is vital in helping them to maintain health and functional independence and lead healthy, independent lives." I wholeheartedly agree with Dr. Moritsugu and am passionate about getting the word out that a healthy eating and fitness plan can have a powerful impact on the quality of their life as they age. As George Burns said, "You can't help getting older, but you don't have to get old."

One of my fitness trainers is a shining example of the difference a healthy lifestyle can make as we age. When I first met Mary, she was my son's high school English teacher. We discovered a mutual love for running and began competing in a few local races together. As I got to know her better, I discovered she had not always been so healthy. She was a smoker and did not participate in much physical activity at all until her mid-forties. When she was diagnosed with painful Trigeminal Neuralgia, her physician encouraged her to find a way to reduce the stress in her life to help manage the pain.

He suggested she try a yoga class, which asks you to focus on your breathing. When the instructor asked Mary to find her breath, she could not, and she knew at that moment she wanted to quit smoking. When she quit, something within her clicked, and she decided it was time for a complete health makeover. She began running, she changed her diet, and, in the process, she found her passion. Mary is now in her 60's and looks not a day over 50.

Mary recently retired after 36 years of teaching. On top of the many volunteer activities in which she is involved, she swims, practices yoga, and runs more than 35 miles a week. When I approached her about the possibility of working with some of my clients as a personal trainer, she took some time to think about it. Then, once she decided that was something she wanted to do, she bought an anatomy and physiology book, made herself a stack of flashcards, got her CPR Certification, and attended Cooper Institute to become a Certified Personal Trainer. Mary is a gifted teacher with a vivacious spirit and contagious smile, but the thing I love most about her is she is an amazing inspiration to my clients who need help believing they can do it.

She is the embodiment of the physical benefits that can come your way when you make the decision to incorporate activity into your life. As you begin a fitness program, two kinds of exercise are equally important in creating a healthy, fit body. The following information will give you the reasons both should be factored into your fitness plan.

Aerobic Training

Investing as little as 30 minutes a day in aerobic activity can add years to your life and improve your quality of life as you age. Aerobics can be defined as brisk physical activity that requires the heart and lungs to work harder to meet the body's increased need for oxygen. Examples of aerobic activities include walking, running, swimming, or cycling performed at a moderate level of intensity that accelerates your heart rate and keeps it elevated for an extended period of time.

During aerobic exercise, you are repeatedly using the large muscles in your body. This causes you to breathe deeper and more rapidly—which maximizes the oxygen in your blood. Your heart will beat faster, which increases blood flow to your muscles and back to your lungs. As your body adapts to regular aerobic exercise, you'll get stronger and you'll burn calories more efficiently.

Before beginning an aerobic training program, do two important things. First, since aerobic training places stress on your heart and lungs, you should check with your physician before beginning a physical training program. Second, start slowly and build up to your goal of at least 30 minutes a day, six days per week. This will give your muscles time to get in condition to handle a more strenuous program.

Some of the specific benefits you will experience from engaging regularly in aerobic training:

Benefit No.1: Chronic disease prevention and management. Aerobic exercise helps combat behavioral diseases such as obesity, heart disease, high blood pressure, type 2 diabetes, stroke and certain types of cancer. And, if you are participating in weight-bearing aerobic exercise, it can help prevent osteoporosis. It helps lower high blood pressure, control blood sugar and can help manage constipation, which seems to be a common complaint as people age. Also, if you've had a heart attack, aerobic exercise can strengthen your heart to help prevent subsequent attacks.

Benefit No. 2: Weight management. Aerobic exercise combined with a healthy eating plan can help you lose weight and keep it off.

Benefit No. 3: Strengthens your immune system. People who participate in regular aerobic training are less susceptible to minor viral illnesses such as colds and flu.

Benefit No. 4: Cholesterol management. Aerobic exercise increases the concentration of HDL (high-density lipoprotein, or "good") cholesterol and decreases the concentration of LDL (low-density lipoprotein, or "bad") cholesterol in your blood, which means less buildup of plaque in your arteries.

Benefit No. 5: Causes endorphins to be released. These are "feel-good hormones" that help fight depression and reduce the tension associated with anxiety. Ever heard of "runner's high?" Blame the endorphins.

Benefit No. 6: Increases your stamina. When you first begin participating in aerobic exercise, you may feel more tired than normal, but over the long term, you'll enjoy increased stamina and reduced fatigue.

Benefit No. 7: Improves mobility and mental sharpness as you age. Aerobic exercise keeps your muscles strong, which can help you maintain mobility. Numerous studies have shown that at least 30 minutes of aerobic exercise three days a week can improve cognitive skills in older adults.

Strength Training

It seems you are in one of two camps when it comes to exercising. You either love aerobics and hate strength training or vice versa. From informal research of simply asking clients which they prefer, they usually say they enjoy aerobic activities more. If you think about it, that makes sense. Aerobic activities are often sports in which participants have some level of competence and finishing produces a release of endorphins, which make us feel great. When you finish your strength training session, if you are like me you just say, "Thank goodness I'm finished with that for one more day." Okay, my bias is showing through, but the point is you probably are going to like one more than the other. Whichever you prefer, you need to make room in your schedule for both. They are equally important in helping you build a strong, healthy body. Strength training comes with its own benefits and is a powerful tool you can use to reduce the signs and symptoms of numerous diseases and chronic conditions.

Benefit No.1: Arthritis Relief. Numerous studies have shown the effectiveness of strength training in the treatment of arthritis. Strength conditioning helps ease the pain of osteoarthritis as well as helping increase muscle strength, improve clinical signs and symptoms of the disease, and decrease physical disability.

Benefit No. 2: Improved Balance. As people age, poor balance and flexibility contribute to falls and broken bones, which can result in significant disability, and, in some cases, death. Strengthening exercises increase a person's flexibility and balance, which decrease the likelihood and severity of falls. A recent study in New Zealand, in women 80 years of age and older, showed a 40 percent reduction in falls with simple strength and balance training.

Benefit No. 3: Increased Bone Density. Strength training has been proven in numerous studies to increase bone density and reduce the risk of fractures. Post-menopausal women can lose 1 to 2 percent of their bone mass annually. Physical conditioning through strength training and weight-bearing exercise is the most proactive step you can take to help counteract this natural occurrence.

Benefit No. 4: Weight Management. Individuals who have more muscle mass have a higher rate of metabolism. A higher metabolism means calories are burned more efficiently. Muscle is active tissue that consumes calories while stored fat uses little energy. Strength training can provide up to a 15 percent increase in metabolic rate, which is enormously helpful for weight loss and long-term weight control.

Benefit No. 5: Improved Glucose Control. America has experienced a 300 percent increase in type 2 diabetes in the past 40 years. One of the most effective means of controlling diabetes can be found by committing to a strength-training program. In a recent study of Hispanic men and women, 16 weeks of strength training produced dramatic improvements in glucose control comparable to taking oral diabetes medication.

Benefit No. 6: Improved Mental State. A good strength-training program can go a long way to lift your spirits. It is not known if this is because people feel better when they are stronger, if strength training produces a helpful biochemical change in the brain, or if it is some combination of the two. What we do know is when older adults participate in strength-training programs, their self-confidence and self-esteem improve, which has a strong impact on their overall quality of life.

Benefit No. 7: Improved Sleep. People who exercise regularly enjoy improved sleep quality. They fall asleep more quickly, sleep more deeply, awaken less often, and sleep longer.

Benefit No. 8: Improved Cardiac Health. Heart disease risk is lower when the body is leaner. The American Heart Association recommends strength training as a way to reduce risk of heart disease and as a therapy for patients in cardiac rehabilitation programs.

Getting Started

Now that you know the benefits of getting your heart pumping and building strong muscle, let's take a look at how to start down a path to a healthier, stronger you. Here are four simple, one-word questions you'll want to answer as you get started:

1. **Who?**—Who in your life will be supportive of your efforts to get healthy and start a workout regimen? It can be a spouse, parent, brother, sister, friend or co-worker. Once you've identified who you can count on for encouragement, make sure to let them know of your plans to get started and then rely on them when you need support. Be aware of the people in your life who may unknowingly try to sabotage your new lifestyle. Change can come hard for some, and the people closest to you may want to keep you just the way you are. Try to love and support them through the changes, letting them know you will still be there for them, even when you are fit, trim and healthy.

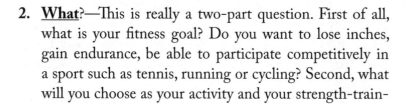

2. **What?**—This is really a two-part question. First of all, what is your fitness goal? Do you want to lose inches, gain endurance, be able to participate competitively in a sport such as tennis, running or cycling? Second, what will you choose as your activity and your strength-train-

ing plan? Do you have a favorite sport? Did you play tennis in high school? Did you run track? Do you enjoy swimming? Do you have friends you could join who belong to a gym? Are you more inclined to participate at home with workout videos? Whatever your choice, take the steps necessary to make them happen—join the gym, buy the videos, dig out your old tennis racket, etc.

My advice on strength training is to hire a personal trainer to get a plan that works best for you. It is more expensive initially, but it can help build your confidence on using weights and keep you from getting injured. Once you have a plan and feel confident that you can maintain good form, you can continue on your own.

_____

_____

_____

_____

_____

_____

3. **When?**—You have to plan your workout into your day— this is key to your success. If you say, "I'm going to start walking 30 minutes a day," but don't plan whether it will be in the morning, at lunch or after work, you will never find time to fit it into your schedule. Your answer to this question will allow you to make a commitment to a time and place where your fitness date will occur every day— no exceptions.

_____

_____

_____

_____

_____

_____

4. **How**?—After your workout, record how you did. It is critical for you to log your progress. Get a journal to track your workouts. It is motivating to look back and see how far you've come. Make note of the date, the time, the activity and leave a column for comments where you can enter how you were feeling, the conditions (if you are training outside), and any other notable information. My husband keeps a great fitness journal. In it he tracks every day's workout along with the statistics on races he has run. He can look back and compare the conditions and the time he ran in a five-kilometer race in 2001 to races this year. It lets him see his progress and keeps him motivated to power on.

_____

_____

_____

_____

_____

_____

I have a website at www.myappetiteforlife.com. I encourage you to visit the site for a variety of helpful tools and links to information that you may find useful as you move toward a balanced life. While you are there, check out some of my favorite healthy recipes, too.

Sticking with It

Sticking with a fitness regimen takes great courage and discipline. Becoming fit will rock your world. Think about it, you've been getting up to work out at 5 a.m. for a year. You've made great strides and seen great results, but it is getting lonely and boring out on that treadmill at 5 a.m. How do you keep motivated to continue? Let me tell you a story of a remarkable young lady who I believe has found the answer to getting started and staying motivated.

My middle daughter, Tabette, grew up in a house with a mom and an older sister who were into health and fitness. Tabette, on the other hand, was this beautifully creative soul who loved to design things—her school projects were amazing and she has always had a great eye for fashion design. She could have cared less about working out or eating healthy. Life to her was to be enjoyed. She has tons of friends, loves to laugh and has always been the life of the party. Growing up she was a little chunky, but she didn't seem to care. She never was able to see the kick in working up a sweat. I tried periodically to encourage her to get involved in physical activities and push away from the table a little sooner, but we love food at our house, and true to her fun-loving spirit, she was more into the pleasure of the moment than self-discipline. Tabette gained a lot of weight, and I know it was hard for her at times. She went to college and had a great time but still had no interest in taking control of her weight.

The summer after she graduated, she had a wonderful opportunity to go to Fisher's Island off the New York coast to be a personal assistant for a woman who lived on the island. She lived on the third floor of this beautiful house and was responsible for shopping, cooking, doing the laundry, and walking the dog. I saw her in April before she left, and then my husband and I went to visit her in late August. When she met us at the ferry, I didn't even recognize her. She had spent the summer shopping on the island for fresh fruits and vegetables, learning to cook healthy dishes, had no access to fast food, and rather than walking the dog, she was running the dog five miles each day. She had done this without saying a word to me, so when Bruce and I were watching for her to get off the boat to pick us up, I had no idea she had totally embraced this new healthy lifestyle.

Tabette is five-feet-two and weighed about 150 pounds when we said goodbye in April. In late August she was down to about 110 pounds and looked amazing. We went with her to run the dog while we were there, and *I* had to ask her if we could slow the pace just a bit. The great news is that was four years ago, and she is still a dedicated runner and healthy eater. She and I have now run three half-marathons together. Occasionally when I go to Austin, I take my running shoes and we scamper along some of her favorite trails around Town Lake. She rides her bike to work, loves to go hiking and spend time outdoors, and truly has fallen in love with an active life. *There it is; did you catch it? The secret to sticking with a fitness plan is this: Build in some variety so you don't get bored, find activities you truly enjoy and keep yourself challenged.*

Tabette's story resonates with many people because this is a society of instant gratification. The majority of us don't want a lifestyle that requires depriving ourselves of the things we enjoy. However, as we mature in our thinking about life, we realize some of the good things we want out of life are going to take a little blood, sweat and tears. I love the fact that in Tabette's renaissance story, she discovered in her own way, in her own time, how to fall in love with fitness. I challenge you to do the same.

"Desire is the key to motivation, but it's the determination and commitment to an unrelenting pursuit of your goal—a commitment to excellence—that will enable you to attain the success you seek."

MARIO ANDRETTI

CHAPTER 5

Overcoming Obstacles

"Health, happiness and success depend upon the fighting spirit of each person. The big thing is not what happens to us in life—but what we do about what happens to us."

FORMER FOOTBALL COACH GEORGE ALLEN

Life is full of hurdles—some a result of choices we've made and some due to circumstances beyond our control. In either instance, we have a choice to make. Will we fall apart or choose joy in the midst of struggle? Will we choose to be a victim of our circumstances or choose to be victorious in the midst of life's painful blows?

We all know people who have suffered great loss; the death of a child or a spouse, a painful divorce, associates diagnosed with terminal cancer. Bottom line, this world can be a painful place. We cannot escape it; it is an inevitable part of life. You've known heartbreak, the kind that knocks the breath out of you and leaves you feeling like you will never be able to continue. Maybe for you it was the harsh words from a spouse saying, "It's over," or a boss calling you in to tell you your services will no longer be needed in a company where you've given the best years of your life, or memories of a painful childhood, or the dreaded phone call that the person you love more than anything has been killed in an accident, or … the list could go on and on.

So here's the million-dollar question:

If heartbreak and sorrow are part of all of our lives, then how can you explain why some people seem so happy and some seem so miserable?

I believe the answer is two-fold. First of all, happy people have chosen to search out and focus on the good things in their lives. By focusing on the positive things, they have disarmed the stronghold of pain and fear that suffering can have on us. This does not mean they are blind to reality; it means they see the good and the bad, and they choose to spend their time focused on the positive. Secondly, those who have found the strength to be happy in the midst of difficult circumstances have learned to be content. Being content is more than just choosing to see the glass half full. It is born out of a heart that trusts God no matter what comes our way. I love this verse in Phillipians where Paul says:

"I know what it is to be in need, and I know what it is to have plenty. I have learned the secret of being content in any and every situation, whether well fed or hungry, whether living in plenty or in want. I can do everything through him who gives me strength."
PHILLIPIANS 4:12-13

Both a positive attitude and contentment are critical to learning to live a life of purpose and joy. Let me give you an example of each:

1. Choosing a Positive Attitude

Recently, there was a flood in Marble Falls, Texas. My mom and her husband have a house there. The house had flooded and they had been up all night bailing water. The water level had risen about two feet on the front of the house, and they had to move all the furniture to the back of the house to keep it from getting wet. It ruined the carpet in the front rooms and they were without water for a couple of days. My son called his grandmother to see how they were doing. She said, "Oh, honey, it's just water. We're fine. It's just 'things' that were ruined, and those can be easily replaced."

My son called me to say, "Why can't Grandma just say, "This is awful; my house is full of water. I'm exhausted; my yard and garden are ruined." The only answer I have is her response to disaster comes from a lifetime of choosing to see the glass half full. She has been counting her blessings in the midst of turmoil for as long as I can remember. Not just in everyday inconveniences, but in hardships and tragedies throughout her life. And, I have to say, as frustrating as that "Pollyanna attitude" can be at times to people like me who can't always pull it off, it is a wonderful Godly heritage for her to give us. I am thankful for a Mom who consistently finds the positive in times of trial and chooses to be joyful or at least at peace with whatever comes her way.

2. Finding Contentment During Tragedy.

For those of us who have had a life experience that completely knocks the wind out of our sails, we know regaining that healthy, happy perspective can be the most difficult thing in the world.

I can't imagine trying to regain focus without Jesus. He tells us this life will have sorrows, but he does not leave us hopeless. In John 16:33, he says, "In the world you will have

tribulation, but take courage; I have overcome the world."
And 1 Corinthians 15:57 says, "but thanks be to God, who
gives us the victory through our Lord Jesus Christ." In Christ
there is hope and victory over defeat. That is a powerful truth
to hang on to when life seems to be crumbling down around
you.

My friend Ruth is a beautiful example of one who has
traveled the road of heartache on a journey to peace and
contentment in the midst of tragedy. She has taught me a
great deal about having the courage to overcome one of life's
cruelest blows. Her 21-year-old son, Luke, left to serve as a
Recon Marine in Iraq in June 2006. He was killed by a road-
side bomb five months later. I've never witnessed that kind of
grief before. Ruth, her husband, John, and their five children
were so close that the loss of their son and brother was almost more than they could endure. It has been many months
now, and watching them all climb out from underneath that
heavy weight of grief and sorrow has been a testimony to
their faith in God and their love for each other.

Ruth has handled this tragedy with her trademark grace
and dignity. She is a strong woman who provides great
strength for her hurting family. But she has also added a re-
freshing component—honesty—to her faith and grieving. I
love that she is so open about her feelings. Grief has many
stages, and Ruth's approach to her feelings will help her move
forward as she slowly continues to heal. She has been very
candid, saying, "I'm angry at God for taking Luke," while in
the next breath clinging to her faith for strength.

Ruth is healing and will survive. She is ready to move
forward to whatever might be next. She is ready to find a
calling, a purpose she feels passionate about. Ultimately, God
has a mighty plan for using her talents and her willing heart

for His glory. I am privileged as her friend to watch His plan unfold.

The process of healing is easier to identify when you are not the one in the middle of it. When you are in the throes of grief and sorrow, it is hard to pull far enough away from it to see what you are going through. It may not be the devastating loss of a child you are dealing with, but if there is something standing between you and a life of joy and purpose, you can take steps to reclaim your zest for living. While many of these steps are difficult, they will ultimately lead you back to a place of peace and contentment in your life.

- Give yourself permission to hurt

  o Loss hurts. It will take time to work through the anger and grief associated with your loss.

- Give yourself time to heal

  o Healing takes time. Don't rush it, but be quick to rely on your faith, your friends and your family for support and strength.

- Find your source of strength

  o This is no time for going it alone. A God-shaped hole can be found in all of us; reach out and allow Him to heal your hurt.

- Accept that change is a part of life

  o Change happens. As we go through different seasons of life, you can count on one thing—change. Some changes are good and some are tragic, but nothing stays the same forever.

- Change your vantage point

- o   Refuse to continue to live in the muck. If tragedy has paid you a visit, take time to hurt, heal, find strength, and then determine to take a fresh look at your circumstances.

- Count your blessings

  - o   Even when darkness surrounds you, begin to identify the blessings in your life. No matter how small they seem, counting your blessings will help change your perspective.

- Look forward

  - o   Do not give in to the temptation to dwell on the past. Fix your eyes on what lies ahead. God gives us a wonderful verse of promise to cling to during times of trial and tragedy: "… weeping may endure for a night, *but joy cometh in the morning.*" Psalm 30:5

- Find your purpose

  - o   You are "uniquely you" because of your experiences. Let God use your individuality to make a difference in the lives of others. As you give your time and energy to help others, you will begin to spend less time thinking about yourself and more time focused on the needs of others. This change of focus will help bring healing.

A part of getting your second wind in life is learning to jump the hurdles placed in our path. Sometimes they are small and seem fairly easy to navigate, but other times they appear to be impossible. What are some hurdles you are facing in your life? Are there obstacles that seem to big too maneuver? Write them down. Next to the hurdle, make a note of how you can jump it. Will it be through changing your attitude, changing your focus, or is it something so seemingly insurmountable that it is only by the grace of God that you will soar over the hurdle? Whatever the answer, don't let your hurdles keep you from getting your second wind. I challenge you to find your way over them. Conquering your hurdles is a big step down your personal path to wellness. The next step is 'Uncovering Your Passion' and you don't want to miss that.

Hurdle: How will I jump it?

_____   _____

_____   _____

_____   _____

CHAPTER 6

Uncover Your Passion

Being passionate is something we all seek. It is your soul's longing. It lights a fire within you and drives you to action. Whether it is the intense chemistry of sexual passion, or the passion that wells up within you when you are worshiping God, or the passion you feel when you have found a purpose that allows you to make a difference in your world;

Passion gives life meaning.

Without passion, life feels like you are simply going through the motions.

If you've not yet discovered the passion in your life that drives you to action, it's time to get off the fence.

Pray for it.
Long for it.
Seek after it.

I have a number of middle-aged women clients and friends who have spent a lifetime taking care of everyone else with little time or energy left to take care of themselves. They've spent the past 20 years juggling kids and all their activities. They've supported their husbands' successful careers. They've done mounds of laundry, cleaned up after everyone, prepared dinner, packed lunches, kissed hurts, and an endless list of other things—many doing all this in addition to holding down a full-time job.

Now the kids have grown up and moved away. The house is quiet, and things stay clean longer. The laundry is next to nothing. Their husbands are busy and they are left to wonder, "What's next?" They feel empty—like their life's purpose is complete, but they have another good 40 to 50 years to live. This can feel devastating, but in reality it is simply a transition into the next wonderful phase of life.

Empty nests are not the only time in life when we experience transition. It happens at all different stages and phases of life: college, marriage, childbirth, divorce, relocating and death of a spouse. The change of season in our lives is just that—change. Depending on your tolerance of change, it may take some time to work through it to find the positive, but when you do, there is a whole big world of joy and excitement waiting for you. Often it is in these times of transition that our quest to find our purpose and passion is born. Everyone needs a life purpose; it gives us a reason to bounce out of bed in the morning ready to tackle the day.

The road to finding your passion takes a different course with everyone—there is no cookie-cutter step-by-step process to arrive at a life of meaning. In fact, I have come to believe that *finding* your passion may be a bit of a misnomer—*I believe your passion evolves.* When you enjoy doing a particular thing, you spend time practicing and perfecting it. As you perfect your skill or talent, others begin to notice how good you are at it. The more others notice your ability, the more you love it, and before you know it, your passion is born.

Let me give you an example to help explain what I'm talking about. My sister-in-law, Terri, has always been the amateur photographer in our family. At holidays and family gatherings, we would rely on Terri to take pictures and send copies to all of us. She is very artsy and photography was something she really enjoyed. She has, for the most part, been a stay-at-home mom and has raised two beautiful girls. One is now a sophomore in college and one is a junior in high school. My brother has a very successful career that takes him out of the country fairly often for weeks at a time. Terri knew she needed and wanted to find her niche. With the girls almost grown and my brother gone a lot, she wanted to find her passion.

Photography was the logical choice for her. It took years of prayer and seeking God for her to discover the passion and purpose she longed for was something she already enjoyed. It was my brother who noticed her natural talent behind the camera. One Christmas he gave her a professional-grade camera. He encouraged her to develop her skill, and the more photographs she took, the more excited she became about pursuing her passion for photography. She continues to attend photography classes at a local community college. She has taken over a spare bedroom and created a state-of-the-art digital imaging and photography studio. I've seen some of her amazing art, and the passion she has for her work shines through. She is now selling her photography and has a very full, rewarding life doing something she loves.

Many of you may identify with Terri's story. It is tough to reach a place in life where you are searching for meaning. If you are wishing you had a map for how to live a life of passion and purpose, then these guidelines may help point you in the right direction.

Top 10 Road Rules to a Life of Purpose:

1. **Map your trip.** Your ultimate destination is to arrive at your passion, that thing in your life that will give you meaning and purpose, but you aren't going to get there in one quick trip. You will need to plan several stopovers— achievable "mini-goals" you can accomplish along the way. And, you know the saying, "the best-laid plans"— don't be surprised or alarmed if plans change midtrip. You are in for the ride of your life.

I remember when I went back to school to focus my efforts on getting into medical school. I was convinced that was the plan God had for my life. I worked very hard to make it happen, but then in mid-stride, the plan changed. I would have never dreamed when I started back to school that I would end up as a dietitian. Now that I am right in the center of what I love doing, I can see how God led me to this very place. One thing is for sure, traveling toward a life of purpose is never dull.

2. **Choose fun travel partners.** Surround yourself with positive people enthusiastic about your journey. This may be family, friends or even new people you meet who share your interests as you explore new avenues.

There is a popular television show right now, The Biggest Loser. While I don't endorse all that they do on the show, I love one thing about it. By the time they get toward the end, when each person in the group has lost close to 100 pounds, they have developed a great camaraderie with each other. They are in a quest toward health and wellness together.

Even though they are competing against one another for the grand prize, they support and encourage each other. In one recent show, the group was asked to do a mini-triathlon in Australia. The two leaders were fighting for first place after a grueling open-water swim, bike ride, and run. The female competitor had been ahead the entire time, but in the end, the guy passed her. He could have won outright, but just before the finish, he chose to wait for her. She carried him across the finish line on her back. When you are working hard to accomplish challenging goals, it is so much more fun and rewarding when you find fun people who are traveling your same path.

3. **Take good road food.** Traveling makes you hungry. Remember, you are not a bystander on this journey. You are going to be actively searching for your passion during this trip and that requires eating foods that will give you energy and a healthy body.

4. **Don't forget to pack your running shoes.** A fit, healthy body will enable you to be strong and ready for action. My husband teases me that the first thing I pack when we are going on a trip is my running shoes. Running on trips does allow me to stay fit, but it is more than that. I love to run in new locations. It gives me a whole new perspective to the area we are visiting. Being on foot allows me to see parks, waterfalls, coffee shops, birds, flowers, people—the things I might otherwise miss if I were flying past in a car.

5. **Travel courageously and with purpose.** Don't be afraid to take some unmarked roads into areas you've never explored. Often the greatest rewards will come from experiences where you have to stretch way beyond what feels comfortable for you. I remember when I began doing on-camera work—I found it exciting, but I hated seeing

and hearing myself on air. It was definitely something that made my heart pound and got my blood flowing, plus I wanted to do it to communicate my message. I knew I wanted to perfect it, but I had to be willing to go down some paths I'd never traveled before to reach the place where I felt comfortable doing live media.

6. **Study places of interest.** As you identify areas of natural interest or ability for you, take time to delve deeper and really explore your God-given talents. You never know, developing one of your natural talents could be the path that leads to your final destination. This is what Terri did when she took time to explore her love of photography. Before long, she was right in the middle of doing what she loves and found her purpose doing that.

7. **Stop and smell the roses along the way.** Your journey to find your passion will have good days and days that seem frustrating. Just like any good road trip, there will be days where you sail effortlessly through hundreds of miles to your next destination, and then there will be those days full of flat tires, overheated engines, and storms that keep you at a standstill. Look at these days as opportunities to slow down and enjoy the journey. You may find blessings where you least expect them.

We live at such a fast pace, it is difficult to slow down. Think about when you get behind someone slow on your morning commute—yikes. I'm not very good at this one, but I do know that the times I've been able to do it, I've have experienced some of the greatest days of my life.

I see lots of patients dealing with cancer. They are usually going through chemotherapy and are coming to see me to try to find a way to cope with symptoms such as extreme nausea, vomiting, dry mouth, and loss of appetite. I make a conscious effort to slow down enough to listen to their story. In listening to them, I am always the one who is blessed. I've learned a lot about being content and finding peace, hope, and even joy in the midst of pain through my cancer patients.

8. **Pack your first aid kit.** When you have experiences that leave you frustrated, feeling discouraged and without hope, you will want to have a good supply of things to bandage you up and make you feel better. Positive self-talk has an incredible impact on the psyche. When things don't go as planned, rather than saying, "I knew I should not have tried this; who am I kidding?" Try saying things like, "I am on a mission, I am strong and determined to learn from this little speed bump and get it right next time." A positive support system can work wonders for keeping you encouraged and on your feet when you hit a bump in the road. Keep in touch with friends and family who can give you a pep talk when you're down. You've claimed God as your source of strength for this journey; now make sure you have a ready list of His promises of strength and support. These will serve to encourage you and keep you energized to pick up and begin again. Here is one of my favorites:

"For I know the plans I have for you," declares the Lord, "plans to prosper you and not to harm you, plans to give you hope and a future."
JEREMIAH 29:11

9. **Use your compass.** On your journey to find purpose, you will encounter many forks in the road that could cause you to lose your way. These may come in the form of

family and friends who don't support your quest, a lack of time, financial barriers and many other challenges that could get in your way. When faced with choices, this verse will be a great compass to help guide you to the right path.

"Finally, brethren, whatever is true, whatever is
   honorable,
whatever is right, whatever is pure, whatever is lovely,
whatever is of good repute, if there is any excellence
and if anything worthy of praise,
dwell on these things."

PHILIPPIANS 4:8

One of the most important ways I've found to stay on course is to listen to my heart. If you start down a path and your spirit seems uneasy, or something about the direction doesn't feel right to you, stop and make the necessary adjustments to get back on track.

10. **If you are there, say "I'm there."** As you are traveling toward finding your passion, be in tune with your soul and listen to your heart—it will tell you when you've reached your ultimate destination. Be alert and ready for action. Finding your life's purpose means it is time to stop the car, put on your work boots, roll up your sleeves, and give it all you've got.

You have arrived.

Finding a life of passion will bring you joy and meaning. Have you noticed when you are in the middle of a project that keeps you focused and energized, you enjoy being alive?

You look forward to tomorrow. You feel like you are contributing, like you are making a difference in your world. I challenge you to take a risk, to dream big dreams, to reach for the stars and be a positive person who leaves a legacy of passion and joy to your world.

CHAPTER 7

Be Engaged

*"A friend is someone who knows the song in your heart
and can sing it back to you when you have forgotten the
words."*

—UNKNOWN

Often when we are searching for our "second wind", we
have experienced something that has separated us from a
close relationship. Whether a divorce, the death of someone
close to you, relocation to a new city, children going off to
college, or any number of other scenarios, getting our second
wind will require the development of new relationships.

Isn't that really one of the deepest longings of our heart?
To have someone know us so intimately they know the song
in our heart and can sing it back to us when we get off track
or lose our way. Friends like that are the people in life who
understand you—your motivations, your fears, your dreams—
and love you anyway.

In a perfect world, we would hope to surround ourselves
with friends we can let get that close to us. However, this
world is far from perfect. Just as joy and good things are a
wonderful part of everyone's life, unfortunately, we all must

handle our own share of pain and suffering as well. Sometimes when difficult circumstances rear their ugly heads, we choose to avoid the pain of life by disconnecting. We choose avoidance to protect ourselves, refusing to feel anything so we don't open ourselves up to hurt and pain.

Finding purpose and passion in life is impossible if you are closed off from your feelings. As you begin breaking down the walls keeping you from connecting with others, you will find life holds a new dimension for you. If you are feeling disconnected, make the changes necessary to re-engage with your world. It can make all the difference between merely living and living a life full of purpose, meaning, and joy.

After going through my divorce, I was single for several years. I dated some, but said openly that I would never re-marry. I had shut myself off from that possibility because I did not ever want to go through that kind of pain again. I had learned to do most things by myself. I bought, remodeled, and sold homes. I did my own yard work. I made a good income—I prided myself in not needing anyone. In fact, when Bruce and I began dating, I made a huge point of making him understand that I didn't need him—I wanted him. I had to slowly learn to trust him enough to let him in close. Now, I have the most amazing husband in the world. He and I are perfectly matched and I am immensely blessed to be sharing life with him. If I had stayed closed off, I would have missed this incredible opportunity to grow old with my soul mate.

Garth Brooks speaks to this in his song, The Dance, where he eloquently describes what we risk if we elect to live life trying to avoid the pain that relationships can bring. He wisely reminisces that he's glad he couldn't see into the future to know how his relationship would end because although he could have missed the hurt, he would have also missed all the good times. His message is a good one for all of us to take to heart: Life is full of good times and trying times, laughter and tears. If we choose to live our lives cautiously to protect ourselves from the pain, we also risk missing the joy.

There is no one right way to be connected to your world. Have you noticed people tend to fall into two major personality groups? Those who seem happy reading, taking a quiet walk either alone or with a close friend. They love to work on projects that don't require large groups of people—like scrapbooking or needlework. Then there are those who live by the motto, "The more the merrier." They are 'joiners'— wherever a group is getting together, they want to be a part. It has taken me a while to understand that both types can be connected to the world around them—some connected to small, intimate circles of friends, and other more gregarious souls connected to a larger group of friends. The point is, in their own way, they are engaged in the world. They have people in their lives with whom they enjoy spending time. They have ties with people whom they love and who love and care about them.

We tend to be quite narcissistic, assuming if someone is different from us, something must be wrong with them. Before we go farther into this chapter, let's make sure of the clear distinction between the well-adjusted people we all have in our lives who prefer either a more quiet or a more boisterous lifestyle, and those building emotional walls to protect themselves from hurt and pain. People use a number of possible barriers to avoid getting emotionally connected with family and friends. If you define fun as going to parties and entertaining a house full of friends and you are married to someone who loves to curl up on the sofa with you and a good book, then you may have some definite compromising to do. It doesn't mean you have deep emotional issues to deal with; it just means you have vastly different interests. You can't change each other, but there are ways to cope, and we will explore some of those later in this chapter.

Have you experienced hurt or rejection that has caused you to emotionally "wall off" your heart and your feelings to avoid ever experiencing that kind of pain again? All of us are capable of disconnecting when we get hurt—the joiners tend to increase the noise going on around them to numb the pain, and the loners tend to pull away until they have no one in their lives to be close to. If you are ready to get your second wind, there may be some walls you've built that need to be torn down. Take a look at this list of invisible walls that may be guarding you from pain ... while keeping you from joy.

- **The wall of busyness.** The person who hides behind busyness is someone who can't be idle; they always have to be going somewhere, doing something. They are active in everything—even things that don't interest them because they are afraid if they slow down they will have to connect with someone.

Excessively busy people often fear that developing a relationship that goes deeper than surface friendliness might require them to let another individual close enough to leave them vulnerable. If you look at your schedule this week, and it is packed 24/7, with no down time, you may need to search your heart to see if you are trying to stay too busy to build a meaningful relationship.

- **The wall of perfectionism.** Are you a person who is compulsive about having everything perfect? Are you afraid of criticism from others if it is not? Do you feel if you keep everything in your life above reproach, you will avoid the pain of someone's disapproval and rejection?

When I began having children, I wanted to have the perfect family. I spent tons of time and energy creating this image of perfection. It was fairly easy with one child, a little more challenging with two, and the leap to three children was too much. Think about it, you have two hands. You can carry two babies, you can put two in the grocery cart, you can fit two car seats in your car, you can hold two hands when crossing the street, but more than that is chaos. By the time I got to four children, all of my hopes for the perfect family were thrown out the window. I know now my need to build this perfect family image was the result of my need to please everyone. I hate to disappoint. Can you relate?

- **The wall of humor.** Are you always making other people laugh in an effort to keep relationships from getting serious? Do you try to keep everyone laughing to avoid meaningful conversation? If so, you may have a fear of rejection. If you fail to make others laugh, people might reject you and not want you around.

- **The wall of anger.** Are you notorious for picking a fight with those who love you in an attempt to keep them at bay? Do you "bark" at family and friends to keep them from getting too close? Are you using anger to manipulate others to keep them at arm's length? Perhaps without anger, you might have to let others in too close. What is the worst that can happen if you let down this protective wall of anger? If you will take a chance, you may just find a soul mate who will share life with you.

- **The wall of escape.** Do you use escape as a means of disconnecting? Spouses often use this one—rather than staying home to work on building a relationship, they elect to escape to a more comfortable place like the golf course, the office, night clubs, or the arms of another. This disconnect is extremely common for people in midlife. It is so subtle and it seems harmless. It can, however, drive a wedge between spouses that is very difficult to remove.

- **The wall of denial.** Are you hiding behind the pretense that everything is fine? You know it is not, but saying everything is great keeps you safe from having to deal with reality. Taking down your guard of denial might mean your would have to endure the pain of dealing with things as they really are rather than seeing life through "rose-colored glasses.

If you can identify with any of these barriers in your life, try to find the courage to take them down—brick by brick if necessary. One of the great things about getting older and having the wisdom of life experiences to draw upon is that you gradually get a little more comfortable in your own skin. I see it as a wonderful gift. I know when I was 30 I really cared what other people thought of me. A lot of choices I made were based on "what would others think," but now at 50 I don't seem to care as much. For example, recently my husband and I went on a long run. It had rained all night, but the rain had stopped and it was extremely hot and humid. After the run, we were hungry for pancakes. We dried off with towels we had in the car, drove to our favorite pancake house and I went in with no makeup, hair pulled back in a ponytail, and semi-dry running clothes. I might as well have gone in screaming, "Look everyone, I'm not perfect." I would have never done that 20 years ago. When you can release your need to hide behind your "wall," you will find a freedom like you've never known. And the best part—as you learn to be yourself, people will be drawn to you for who you really are. No more hiding.

A tragic result of building barriers that disconnect you is a lack of emotional intimacy. This can happen in all stages of life, but is often most visible in marriages as the kids are graduating from high school and leaving home to begin lives of their own. Couples have spent the past eighteen years with their relationship revolving around who is taking Johnny to his baseball game and who is driving Sally to ballet. The weeks, months and years fly by while they just try to keep their heads above water juggling all the activities. By staying busy with the kids, there is often no time or energy left to connect with each other. As the household slows down and the husband and wife are left to figure out how to reconnect, there can be some trying times ahead.

One of the most common complaints among married couples in midlife is that they feel they are just going through the motions. They desperately miss the emotional intimacy of sharing their hopes and dreams with someone who knows them completely and loves them anyway. This can be a dangerous time in the relationship. Spouses might find they have grown so far apart that another person or activity becomes more appealing than honoring the commitment they made to each other to work together and grow together through tough times.

If you can work through this stage of life, you, your spouse, and your family will come out much stronger and more solid than ever. As with most life challenges, communication is the key to success. Take time to envision what your "post-children" years will look like to you. I've listed some topics and questions below to help you begin some introspection on what you'd like to do. If you are married, ask your spouse to do the same thing, and then compare answers. Be sure to include an honest evaluation of your health, your fitness level, and your outlook on life to see if the lifestyle you are dreaming of can become reality.

This simple activity may go a long way toward helping avoid conflict down the road. Keep in mind there are no right or wrong answers to these questions, but you and your spouse may answer them differently. The purpose of sharing your answers with each other is to open the lines of communication and avoid unrealized expectations and potential conflict down the road. Find time to sit down together to share. This might be a perfect chance to schedule a weekend getaway specifically designed to help draw you closer together. Sitting on a blanket at the beach sharing a glass of wine may be the perfect setting to disarm the tension and allow you both the freedom to share your hopes and dreams with each other.

Planning for the Second Half:

- How I see my typical day—go through each segment of the day from waking to sleeping

- Things I want to do together

- Things I want to do with friends

- Things I want to do alone

- Hobbies I enjoy and those I plan to cultivate

- Plans to work part-time or volunteer

- Ways I plan to make a difference in my world

- Things I'd like to achieve

- Places I'd like to go

- People I'd like to visit

- Major purchases I'd like to make

- Plans to further my education

When my husband and I were dating, we enjoyed doing everything together. He played tennis, so I was learning to play. I love to run, so he ran with me. Every Saturday we would go for a long run and then go to breakfast. The week we returned from our magical honeymoon in Hawaii, Saturday morning came, and he announced he was leaving to go play tennis. I was crushed. I assumed our Saturday mornings were sacred. After we talked about it, I understood Saturday mornings were when his new San Antonio league played, and that was very important to him to help him make new friends (he relocated to San Antonio with me when we married). It was not that he didn't want to spend time with me; it was simply a breakdown in communication. If we had taken the time to cover some of the questions I listed above before we tied the knot, we might have avoided the hurt feelings.

Staying connected can be especially challenging if you are single or if you are relocating to a new area away from family and friends. The U.S. Census Bureau reported in 2005 that close to 90 million unmarried and single people were living in America. Of those, almost 15 million were age 65 and older. Many times, recently widowed spouses will relocate to be closer to family, so they have the compounded challenge of being newly alone and newly relocated. Some reports indicate that as many as 59 percent of Americans will relocate at retirement. These are staggering statistics and important to consider as we discuss staying engaged in a life of purpose and meaning.

When you are alone in a new location, it takes effort to get involved and build a circle of friends. It sounds almost trite to say, "Find groups of people who have similar interests and become an active member." It may be trite, but it really is sound advice and can be a good avenue for meeting new people. Another piece of advice is to find people who need something you have to offer and to get involved. After my uncle died tragically from an inoperable brain tumor, leaving my aunt a widow in her late 50s, she found a wonderful way to stay connected. My Aunt Mike (this is not a typo, 'Mike' is short for Michelle) is an accomplished musician. She sings and plays piano and the pipe organ beautifully. She found a start-up church in Santa Fe, N.M., that needed a pianist, and she offered to play. Needless to say, they loved her and she grew to love them. It was a blessing to her to be able to share her gift, and it was an amazing blessing to those for whom she played.

> *Friendship doubles our joy and divides our grief.*
> —SWEDISH PROVERB

As your life changes seasons, you will walk through times where you must purposely, actively cultivate new friendships and find new people with whom to connect. Let me tell you about my mom. When my father became ill, she and my dad moved backed to the states after living in Panama for several years. Mom loves church and her life revolves around being active in a variety of areas of service there—everything from singing in the choir, to attending women's Bible study groups, to teaching Sunday school, to volunteering with mission groups. When they moved to Lubbock, she was busy caring for my father during his illness. When he passed away, she began searching for ways to get more involved.

Part of her activity was to help fill the void of missing my dad, but a greater part was that active is who she is and "church" is what she wants to be doing. In addition to her work at the church, she loved inviting people over; neighbors, married couples, and widows. She organized block parties in her neighborhood. Soon she had made several new friends who were inviting her to dinner, to the symphony, to parties, and to girls' weekend getaways. The point is this: she recognized getting engaged in her world and staying connected was important to her health and happiness. She also recognized that making a connection as a newly single person in a new city would require effort from her. She was willing to make the effort and it paid big dividends.

I'll never forget when my brother and I threw a big 70th birthday party for her in the church parlor a few years later. We asked her for a list of people she wanted to invite. She gave us a big list of new friends as well as some longtime friends who lived a few hours away. I remember her saying to us, "You are so sweet to do this, but what if no one comes?" Needless to say, the place was packed. Friends came from miles around. She has that wonderful gift of giving herself away to everyone she meets. She is positive, pleasant and fun to be around. She has boundless energy and a contagious spirit. Her life is a beautiful template for those seeking to get connected.

Plant a seed of friendship; reap a bouquet of happiness.
—LOIS L. KAUFMAN

One of the best things about becoming engaged with others in relationships is it enriches the lives of both parties. If you are looking for a friend and make the effort to reach out, then each of you has received a blessing. Intimate friendships must be nurtured and they take time to unfold. As you become involved in groups of people, there will be some in the group who you will get to know as friendly acquaintances. These relationships are fun, but they usually stay on the surface. However, you will find one or two in the group with whom you can make a deeper connection, the kind of friends you can share your feelings, fears and personal struggles with. A friendship like that takes commitment and work from both sides. A good friend understands you and loves you just the way you are, and you do the same for them. When you find a friendship like that—you have found a treasure.

"A friend is a gift you give yourself."
—ROBERT LOUIS STEVENSON

As you journey toward tearing down emotional walls that have kept you from connecting with people, I want to challenge you to take a risk. This book is all about finding the courage to make changes that will enrich your life. Reach out to someone and be the friend they need. Reach out to your spouse each day and take the time to nurture the special relationship you share. Find a gift or talent you have and share it with others. Spend more energy thinking about what you can do to enhance the lives of those around you than about how lonely and mistreated you are. As the famous quote by Ralph Waldo Emerson says,

"The only way to have a friend is to be one."

CHAPTER 8

Take a Stand: Be Confident

*You've got to take the initiative and play your game. In a decisive set, **confidence** is the difference.*

—CHRIS EVERT

Confidence rises from the inner assurance that you are capable and competent to meet any circumstance and handle it. It blossoms when your physical, mental, and emotional health is optimum, and you know you are at your best. Taking the initiative to get healthy has a tremendous impact on your confidence. Choosing health takes courage and it takes hard work. As you experience noticeable progress in your quest for health, you will feel a sense of accomplishment and pride. Investing in your body by nourishing it with deliciously healthy foods, getting fit through activities that build strength and muscle, and determining to find and enjoy the good things in your life, brings with it the unexpected bonus of a super boost in confidence.

I had a weight-loss client who described this phenomenon perfectly. He said, "When I was at my heaviest, I would see things around the house that needed to get done, but I thought... I'll do that later. Now that I've lost 30 pounds, I see things that need to be done around the house, and I go ahead and tackle them." I often hear comments similar to that, and I know their call to action is partly from an increase in energy, but I also know once people start taking control of one area of their lives, they suddenly begin to feel confident that they can successfully take on other areas as well.

To discover your own "confident" self; it's as easy as
Take 3—*Taking the First Step, Taking a Risk, and Taking Charge.*

Take the First Step:

I believe a lot of people in this world planned to live a life much different than the one they are living. Life has a way of taking twists and turns that can throw us off balance. If you lose your footing and begin making poor choices, before you know it, you are in a mess. It's really odd, but you actually get out of a mess the same way you got in. You take a stand and say to yourself, "From this moment forward I resolve to make choices that are good for me." You can't change everything at once, but by beginning to reverse the downward spiral—determining to make wise choices to improve in one area—you begin to feel more powerful, more in control of your life. Once you make one good choice, the next one seems a bit easier to make, and it snowballs from there. The toughest part is the first step.

I hired a young assistant who had completed some college and had fallen into the trap so many do, financing many things without adequate income in place to pay them off. She got so far behind on her payments that it didn't seem possible to ever catch up. Creditors were calling her all the time. She was also making poor choices in other areas of her life. She lived on fast food, made friends with people who partied too hard, and formed relationships with people who did not have her best interest at heart.

When she came to work for me, she began to hear the message of health, hope and happiness we share with our clients. I think she may have been a bit skeptical at first, but she eventually started making small, significant changes in her life. She began running and doing some strength training. She started eating healthier and partying less. She has begun slowly but surely, paying off some of her debt. It was as if taking the stand to get healthy gave her the confidence to take control in other areas of her life. She was able to get a car and signed up to begin taking classes to complete her degree. The confidence that stems from reclaiming control over your life is empowering. It gives you the courage to create the life of purpose and meaning you've always imagined for yourself.

Take a Risk:

The things we desire in life often seem just out of reach. To get there, you have to take a chance and step out in faith. I had the opportunity several years ago to take a risk and pursue my dream. By stepping out of my comfort zone, I found a career that exceeded my wildest expectations.

I had been working as a dietitian at Methodist Hospital in Lubbock, Texas for about two years when I attended a national dietetics conference. One of the breakout sessions was led by Lori Valencic, a supermarket dietitian from Houston. She was sharing how she got into that particular specialty, and I found her story fascinating. I spoke with her afterward, and she said, "If you are in Lubbock, you should approach United Supermarkets to see if they would be interested in hiring a Corporate Dietitian." I went home and couldn't get the idea out of my mind. I thought about it, prayed about it, and decided to go for it. I put together a proposal, contacted someone I knew at the company and found that I should present my idea to Dan Sanders, who at that time was Chief Marketing Officer at United. I had a great meeting with Dan, and he invited me back to interview with a couple of other people. Ultimately, they offered me the job. It was the chance of a lifetime.

I was getting a huge increase in pay, a car, and tons of perks that come with taking a job in the corporate world. Other than the one-hour conversation with the dietitian from Houston, I had no idea what a Corporate Dietitian did for a supermarket chain. And, this was a new position that I had proposed to United, so the company wasn't sure what to do with me, either. Luckily, I love paving new trails, so I found it very exciting. They gave me a short "honeymoon period" to become familiar with the industry, and then I began the most challengingly wonderful years of my life. They basically said, "Here is your office. Make us proud."

I was able to create my job—to do what I thought a dietitian would do in my position. I wrote articles for ad circulars and created an in-store recipe card program—even managing the food photography, recipe card design, and working with a fixture specialist to design the in-store unit to display the cards for customers. I was at United as the natural, organic craze was evolving, so I was able to create a health-food section for the stores. I was there just as the big buzz began in the industry about "Home Meal Replacements." I had the opportunity to work with a fixture company to design a refrigerator-freezer unit for stores to house the ingredients needed to make the recipe of the week. When United decided to bring ready-to-eat meals to its delis, I was on a team that developed the recipes. I was promoted to Director of Consumer Solutions, which meant my last few years at United were spent as part of a team that flew across the country examining exciting new trends in the food industry. We would then bring the best ideas back and find a way to implement them in our new concept Market Street stores.

This story shows the transformation that can come from confidence. At my low point after my divorce, I would have never had the confidence to pull that off. I was tired. I was defeated. But I knew I wanted more. I knew I didn't want to grow old and die thinking what a mess I'd made of my life. I was at the bottom of a deep, dark well and could barely see the light from above. I still believe to this day that I found the courage and the energy to step toward the light because of the prayers of my family and friends, and particularly, my mom.

If you've ever gone through a dark time in your life, you will identify with this.

Looking back, you can see God's hand carrying you toward the light—one small step at a time. When you are in the middle of it, you are questioning every decision you make and frantically seeking God's direction in your life. It is hard to see until you are close enough to the top to look back and see that God prepared the way and directed your path all along.

After making the decision to pick up the pieces and start again, I had lots of work to do to get my second wind. I knew I wanted to get healthy so I started running and changed my diet, I wanted to be a good mom, so I spent more quality time with my kids. I wanted my life to count for something, so I finished my degree and found ways to give back to my community. Little by little these efforts added up, and I was being transformed into a capable, confident person. I put in two years of hard work at the hospital, learning to apply the knowledge I had acquired in school. I felt competent as a dietitian. The cumulative effect of all these small successes led me to believe I could pursue loftier goals. When the opportunity of a career in corporate dietetics presented itself, I had the confidence to take a risk. The reward for me was a dream job that absolutely rocked my world. The experience at United was so much more than I could have ever imagined. When you trust God for the courage to take a chance, it could be the thing that redirects the rest of your life.

> *Blessed is the man who trusts in the Lord and has made the Lord his hope and confidence.*
> —JEREMIAH 17:7

Take Charge:

Is it time for you to take charge of your life? Are there things that must change for you to enjoy the health and happiness you desire? You can take steps to build your self-confidence and get a jump-start on feeling good about yourself and your abilities:

1. Reflect on past accomplishments. Make a list of the top five to ten accomplishments you are most proud of in your life. Identify what strengths you used and what circumstances contributed to your success. Bask in the glory of what you achieved; allow the feelings to be the foundation of your budding self-confidence.

2. Take stock of your natural abilities. If you're stumped, think about what your friends and family would consider as your strengths.

3. Pick some low-hanging fruit. Find something where you are sure to be successful and start with that. Successes—even small ones—build confidence.

4. Set goals that allow you to shine. Maximize your strengths and minimize your weaknesses.

5. Practice positive self-talk. Build a strong arsenal of personal mantras that will help encourage you to stay strong when you feel like quitting.

6. Educate yourself. Become a student of the area where you'd like to excel—learning everything you can that will make you more knowledgeable in your area of expertise. Identify the skills you'll need to achieve your goals. Don't take shortcuts. Becoming the best at the goals you've set for yourself may mean some short-term sacrifices. It may mean taking college courses, completing an internship, or taking an entry-level job to study with someone you admire. All these things may seem to slow you down; they will ultimately allow you the success you desire.

7. Be committed to excellence. Success is hard work. The people you know who are successful and self-confident have worked much harder to get there than you may ever know. How hard are you willing to work? To achieve excellence, you have to discipline yourself to drive tirelessly toward your goal.

8. Learn to handle failure. Accept that mistakes happen when you're trying something new. Look at mistakes as learning experiences. There is no how-to manual on life. Even though you have planned well, taken time to get educated, and worked really hard to make wise choices, you will experience failure. They are a part of life that

teaches us more about ourselves than any success ever will. Failures build character, and ultimately that is the most important quality anyone can possess.

9. Stretch yourself. Initially, you want to select goals you know you can reach easily. As your confidence grows, challenge yourself. Set bigger goals—goals that take you out of your comfort zone.

While there are a multitude of things we can do to actively pursue confidence, the reality of life offers additional paths to confidence, but you definitely have to pay your dues to travel them.

Walking through heartache:

When you have one of those life experiences that brings you to your knees, the pain can be quite humbling. But as you muddle through doing the best you can, you achieve this odd sense of confidence that says, "Wow, if I handled that, I'm pretty sure I can handle anything that comes my way."

About 10 years ago, I had the most humbling experience of my life. Even now, as I am writing these words, it is very difficult for me to be this open. While it is something I'd rather keep secret, I know many families out there are suffering private pain from similar experiences. My daughter and I both hope and pray that by sharing this story with you, you will find God's mercy and grace to make it through situations and circumstances you are dealing with.

Our story:

When my youngest daughter was 15, she came running downstairs in the middle of the night crying. She flopped herself on my bed and said, "Mommy, I'm pregnant." I kept trying to reassure her that she was just having a bad dream. She could not be quieted. We sat on the bed talking, and I realized I might be the one having a bad dream. Long story short, she was pregnant, and our lives were about to be turned upside down. A trip to the doctor the following day revealed that she was almost five months pregnant. Of course, I went through the guilt of trying to figure out how I could have missed all the signs. And, I know this sounds shallow, but I was embarrassed, and a pregnant teenage daughter is hard to cover up.

Abortion was not an option either of us could consider, so we decided to pull her out of school and put her in another city at an adoption center where she could finish the spring semester of her sophomore year. That lasted about three weeks. She did not like being away from home, and I missed her terribly, so I picked her up and brought her home. We considered having her attend an alternative school in our city, but that didn't seem a good option for her, either. Ultimately, we went back to her high school, met with her principal, Dr. Mike Bennett, and it is a meeting neither of us will ever forget. Dr. Bennett looked right at my daughter and he was so gracious. He said, "You are an amazing young lady. You have ended up in a very difficult situation, and you are facing it head on. You are a Monterey Plainsman, and your place is here with your friends and classmates. We want you here, and if I can ever do anything to help, you let me know."

His kind words were an oasis of acceptance in a desert of raised eyebrows. We left there with newfound hope and courage. That evening, I gave myself "a good talking to." I reflected on the strength of the women in my life. I thought about my mom's mother. My grandmother could hoe cotton with the best of them. She moved water pipes in the fields;

she planted huge gardens, canned fruits and vegetables tire-lessly, and was truly an amazing woman.

Then there is my dad's mom who came through the Great Depression, working in the shipyards during the war. She was strong and sure. And you've already heard stories about my mom. She is the most amazing woman ever. She is gracious and kind. She is smart and can work harder and with more energy than anyone I've ever known. As I thought about all the strong women in my life, I thought, "Jan, you come from a long line of very strong women, and you can handle this."

The next day, I could hardly wait to share the message with my daughter. We had certainly been humbled by the situation, and the humility we were feeling had stripped us of all our pride. It left us in a very raw, but teachable state. I truly believe God gave me that message of strength and hope at just the right time—when we so desperately needed it. We found power and courage in those words. That personal mantra of strength and the reminder of our God-given abil-ity to handle anything that comes our way carried us through the next few months. The pregnancy, the birth of a precious little girl, and the bittersweet adoption to a wonderful Chris-tian family all was heavier than anything we could have en-dured on our own, but God is good. He gave us His strength and the reminder of our heritage of strength. It's funny, but we still use that mantra on each other today. If I am going through a tough time, my daughter will call or send me a card saying, "Remember, Mom, you come from a long line of very strong women. You can handle this."

Confidence is the sure footedness that comes with
having proved you can meet life.

—ANN LANDERS

Celebrating Birthdays:

Another confidence-builder is getting a certain number of birthdays behind you. As we approach the second half of life, something wonderful happens. (So do a lot of really awful things like droopy skin, gray hair, and menopause, but let's try to stay positive). With a few years of life under your belt, you gain wisdom. You've experienced quite a lot of life and have learned some valuable, sometimes painful, lessons. One of the best lessons is you are a person of value and worth—warts and all—not because of your own perfection, but because of who God is in your life. You no longer feel the need to make people like you more by pretending to be something you are not. You have grown comfortable in being exactly who you are, and you revel in being your "authentic self." That is confidence. I find people who have mastered the art of being at home in their own skin some of the most fascinating, approachable, beautiful people I know—regardless of their outward appearance.

Developing confidence in who you are—the good, the bad, and the ugly—is one of the most important secrets to living a joy-filled life. Confidence brings a poise and self-assuredness to which others are drawn. Think of the people you admire. Do they have perfect skin and flawlessly toned bodies? Or, are you drawn to people with wide smiles, who hold their head high and live with purpose and meaning? Confident, self-assured people tend to take better care of their physical, mental and emotional health. They recognize they are at their best when they eat healthy, keep their bodies fit, and concentrate on seeing the good in themselves because they know they are worth it.

I once had a client who was a competitive swimmer. Upon entering high school, he consulted with me because he was a little overweight. Actually, he was just a little short for his weight—his height needed a chance to catch up. His mom brought him in to make sure they were doing everything they should be to give him the nutrition he needed to be at his best. I made a few suggestions, and he was open to making the changes. I challenged him by saying, "You are starting fresh this school year. It's a new year in a new school. You are a very talented swimmer and have a lot going for you. Why not reinvent yourself into an athlete who doesn't put junk into your body? People respect that. It says to those around you, 'I honor my body by fueling and training it to be the best it can be.' That is a cool thing to be known for."

He took my challenge, will you?

The height of your accomplishments will equal the depth of your convictions.

—WILLIAM F. SCOLAVINO

Chapter 9

Age Gracefully

A giant step toward getting your second wind and making a fresh start is determining to age gracefully. Aging brings with it a unique set of challenges—illness, loneliness, loss of energy and mobility, death of friends and family—just to name a few. The way your body operates changes dramatically. You need fewer calories as you age, your metabolism slows, your muscle mass decreases, and you have to work harder at staying fit. Your vision begins to fade, and reading the newspaper can be an impossible task without your "cheaters" on. Your skin begins to lose its firmness, and gravity begins to take effect, leaving you with wrinkles and creases where none existed before. The things we once counted of utmost importance—our looks and our functionality—are slowly deteriorating, and regardless of how hard we work at staying "young-at-heart," ultimately we feel powerless to do anything about this natural progression of life.

There are three components of healthy aging that I believe have a huge impact on our ability to age gracefully. The first two are good nutrition and physical activity which we have talked about extensively in previous chapters. No doubt good nutrition and physical activity will help slow the natural decline that happens as we age. The benefit of practicing a healthy lifestyle is to avoid, or at least slow, the deterioration that results from poor health practices and bad lifestyle choices. Todd Whitthorne, President of Cooper Concepts, a division of The Cooper Clinic in Dallas, Texas, calls it "squaring off the curve." As he puts it, "The goal in life is to live every day to the fullest, having the health and energy to enjoy a full life. Then, one day when you've reached a ripe old age, you just get sick and die." What Todd is saying is regardless of how hard we try, our bodies will still eventually grow old and die. It is part of life. Through a healthy lifestyle, we can square off the typical downward curve of decline. The curve that often begins at midlife and continues at a fairly rapid decline until the quality of life we are living is compromised, and we are no longer living a vibrant, active life. This curve of decline often ends with your last years spent in a nursing facility, unable to perform even the simplest activities of daily living. By making healthy choices in diet and exercise, we square off the curve, living a rich, full, active life until the end.

You've seen the bumper sticker, and it's true:

GROWING OLD—IT AIN'T FOR SISSIES.

I've painted a pretty bleak picture in this chapter so far, but I've done so purposely. I want to help you see the importance of the third and arguably the most important component of healthy aging. If you've built your self-worth and your life's meaning around your appearance and your abilities, the aging process can leave you feeling desperate and without value. The frailty of life and the inevitability of death can leave us with nothing to hold on to as we grow old if all our worth has been built on fleeting things such as youthful beauty and fitness. So the question is this: How do we equip ourselves to lead a healthy active life while finding peace and fulfillment throughout our life cycle? The powerful third component is getting in touch with your very core and connecting with a trusted friend or life partner and with God.

We all have inside of us a soul, an essence of spirit, that makes us unique. It is the quality that draws us to connect with each other. Tragically, some of us have spent lots of time and energy trying to be someone we thought others wanted us to be and not being true to our authentic self. It is impossible to connect on the deepest level with someone who is not real. This part of the aging process is especially difficult for people still pretending to be something or someone they are not. The longer we pretend, the more challenging it becomes to uncover the core of who we really are. Getting in touch with your core—determining who you are, what drives you, what is important to you, what you are passionate about, what you enjoy—is the third component of healthy aging that will bring you joy and fulfillment throughout the process.

Though I have certainly rebelled against it at times in my life, I have come to realize the thing that drives me and keeps me grounded is faith. According to the lyrics of a song, "There's a God-shaped hole in all of us..." To me, that means God created us each with a void, a place that can only be filled by Him. I have tested and tried that theory and have found it to be true. I have an innate need to connect with God. Without faith in something greater than myself, I can easily become wrapped up in my own unmet needs and the inequities in my life. I become miserable—and miserable to be around.

Studies have shown repeatedly those who report a happy, fulfilled life as they age are those who have a deep, abiding relationship with God. For me, connecting with a belief system that is greater than my own meager existence helps make sense of life, death and everything in between. As I have recognized my need for God and built my life around developing a relationship with Him, He has been faithful to be my source of strength and comfort throughout the ups and downs of life.

Nothing brought this reality home to me more than the death of my father. As I've shared previously, 1994 was a difficult year for my family and me. When my dad lost his battle with cancer in August that year, it seemed like the cruelest blow of all. I wasn't sure how I was going to make it through life without him. I've always been a "daddy's girl." I was only 37, and because of everything else going on in my life I really needed to rely on his strength and wisdom.

My children loved being around my dad. My mom and dad represented strength and stability to them while almost everything else in their young world seemed to be falling apart. My father began showing some concerning symptoms while he was in Panama. By the time he got to the states and was diagnosed with prostate cancer, it had already spread to his lungs, so the prognosis was not good from the start of his treatment. However, we hoped, prayed, and trusted God for a miracle until the very end.

When Dad died, I dealt with a lot of anger and resentment toward God for taking away the one safety net the kids and I had. It took me from August to Easter of the following year to find peace. I'll never forget the evening I crawled into bed and these words just came pouring out of me. I had to get up and write them down. I believe God gave me the words to this poem to bring healing to my heart. On Easter in 1995, my children, my mom, my dad's mother and I went to my father's grave, and I read this poem to my family:

A Tribute to My Father
Wade Hampton (Jack) Pearce, Jr.
1927-1994

I never thought I'd make it without you to guide and
comfort me.
I trembled at the thought of being alone.
You know me, I questioned God's good judgment at
taking you
When my children so desperately needed a man to
look up to, and
When I so needed to lean on your wisdom and
strength.
Things are so hectic down here, Dad.
I don't know how we'd make it without Mother.
She brings us calm and serenity
In the midst of our chaos, and
We receive it as a priceless gift.
She is quite a treasure, and I know you miss her.

So often I wish for you to be back with us whole and
healthy again.
Your absence has left a gaping hole in our lives.

But, the real tribute to you is
We are making it on our own.
You taught us well the
Source of Strength and Companionship
You taught us perseverance for the task at hand.
You taught me to relish life, and not to fear death.

I am uniquely me because of who you dared to be
Thank you for instilling in me the ability to carry on
     during life's most difficult trials.
Thank you for believing in me, and teaching me to
     believe in myself.
Thank you for teaching me that I am more than a
     conqueror through Him who loves me.

Once I was able to pen those words and read them aloud to my family, I was able to make peace with my father's death. As I said earlier, I have tested and tried my need for God. I think accepting God's love and His omnipotence is easier for some than for others. The great truth that I have finally accepted is this: God created me to be exactly who I am. He knows my natural tendency is to bow up against things I perceive to be unfair or unjust.

That same "fight" within me is the part of my personality that makes me an effective warrior against destructive behavior like gorging on junk food and being a couch potato. I used to hate my feisty spirit, and I spent lots of my life trying to squelch it, thinking it was ungodly. But with maturity and the grace of God, I've been able to view it from a different perspective. I've come to understand a maverick spirit is the quality within me that breeds "creative perseverance." It draws me to question, doubt, and struggle through problems until I come to some kind of personal resolution on the issues and circumstances that come my way.

Perhaps you are thinking, "That sounds just like me," or maybe you have similar struggles with some strong personality trait. The good news is God made you just the way you are. Quit fighting within yourself to be something you're not. Be real and watch God use your perceived "flaw" for His glory. My father had a very strong personality, and, shall we say, "I am very much my father's daughter." My ex-husband actually has a great line he used to say about me—"I thought I was marrying Ganelle (my sweet, always appropriate, gracious mom), but instead I got Jack." That's okay. God used my dad in a mighty way to bring the good news of Jesus to people all over the world. I'll gladly follow in his footsteps.

As you test boundaries and scrape to get to the core of who you really are, I want to encourage you. Regardless of what you find, don't mask it. I've come to understand that questioning, exploring, trying, and failing is an important part of getting in touch with your true essence. Identifying who you are and understanding God loves you as you are, that he created you to be that way, and learning to accept yourself is paramount to finding peace in your life.

What does it mean to find your core?

In fitness training, when you work to develop core strength, you are working to strengthen your abdominal and back muscles, the ones that hold the rest of you upright. In spirituality, it means getting in touch with your innermost self. It means drilling down into your soul until you clearly see what drives you, what fuels your dreams and passions. Getting in touch with this core will guide you toward living the life you've always dreamed.

How can you find your core?

Awakening to the awareness of who you are is not something that happens overnight. Finding your core can be compared to being pregnant with your first child. It is an exhilarating series of experiences full of excitement, joy, pain, and a host of other emotions. You've heard others explain their pregnancy experience, but until you've actually walked through the full nine months for yourself, you have no idea what to expect. This unique little human being inside you grows and develops day by day. When this precious one decides it is time to enter the light of day, the experience for mom is often one of the most difficult things she will ever go through. But, ask anyone who has ever given birth, when you first hold the life that was created and grew inside you for nine months, the result was worth every moment of temporary discomfort.

Just like childbirth, giving birth to your true essence takes time, patience, and perseverance. But the result is worth the effort. The birthing process you must go through to open the door to your soul is the key to finding peace, contentment, and fulfillment.

Getting to the C.O.R.E. of who you really are:
    C = Connect
    O = One—embrace time alone
    R = Reach Out
    E = Enjoy

Connect. First of all, make a connection with God. He promises in his word (Jeremiah 29:13) that, "You will seek Me and find Me when you search for Me with all your heart."

There are many ways you can begin your search for Him. Pray. Ask God to make Himself real to you. Read your Bible, praying as you read that God would give you understanding. Ask a friend who attends church if you can go. Tune your radio station to Christian music. As you make the first step toward searching for God, He will surround you with His love and His grace like you've never known.

Secondly, make a connection with someone special. Soul mates are not found, they are forged over time through sharing tiny glimpses of your soul with another trusted soul. Dare to fall in love. If you are married, start with your spouse. I know that sounds funny, but it seems that many couples grow apart as they age. It's not that they don't love each other, but the busyness of life has taken them in different directions. All of a sudden, they look up, they've been married for thirty years, and they have nothing in common. These are the people you see in restaurants who sit down, eat, pay, and leave without ever making eye contact or saying a word to each other. If the love connection between you and your spouse has been severed, it's time to make some drastic changes.

- Be a person someone would want to spend time with.

    o Take care of yourself. Remember what you did when you were dating? You took a shower, did your hair, put on your makeup, and wore your nicest clothes so that you could look your best. Think how you would feel if your spouse did this for you.

    o Court your spouse. Make his/her favorite meal. Leave a sweet note on his/her pillow. Put a bag of M&M's in his/her briefcase (that is what my husband does for me when I travel). Actually, my husband is a master of "little surprises." The other day, I mentioned this new musical artist I really liked. I told Bruce I had been listening to her songs on the Internet. A few days later, we were cleaning up the kitchen after dinner. I picked up the dishtowel and underneath he had left a copy of her CD. I can't tell you how that small act of kindness filled me with joy and excitement.

o   Be happy. You've got a choice to make when it comes to your attitude. There is an old saying, "You can be right, or you can be happy." Most of the time it is just not that important in the grand scheme of things to get someone to admit you are right. If you are right, be right, with no need to be smug or beat the issue to death trying to win a petty argument. Put a smile on your face and spread a little joy. Take a look at your life. You can find something to be happy about.

-   Find a trusted friend. The world is full of people who want to be loved and feel the need to be connected, just like you. Join groups that enjoy the same things you do—if you like to crochet, then find a needlework shop close to you and join one of their groups. If you run, join the local running club. Find a church you enjoy and get involved. Within the groups you join, look for the one or two people with whom you could really build a deeper relationship, and then take a risk—be a friend to them first and see what happens.

-   Consider a pet. Go to your local animal shelter and find a four-legged friend to love. There are so many homeless animals who, with a little love and attention could be a loyal, trusted companion for you. They don't take the place of human relationships, but scientific studies have shown repeatedly that a beloved pet can add years to your life.

-   Try online. You have to use judgment, common sense, and discretion, and even then, online dating may not be for everyone. But, I know personally of many success stories. In this day and time when every second of the day is packed full of work and family responsibilities, little time exists to meet someone special. Bruce and I have several friends who have found this to be a fun and successful way to meet that person. We've hosted two weddings at our home of friends who met through a Christian online dating service.

For example, let me tell you another story about my Aunt Mike. After my uncle died, she spent several years alone, then one day a fun, crazy friend of hers came to her home and said, "You are too young and too beautiful to spend the rest of your life alone. I'm going to help you set up a profile on e-Harmony." At first my Aunt protested, but it turned out to be fun. She met some really nice people, and ultimately, she met and married a fabulous man who had lost his wife in an automobile accident a few years before. They now live in a beautiful home on the Outer Banks of North Carolina and are having a wonderful time sharing life together. If she had not been willing to take a risk to do something totally out of character for her, their paths might never have crossed.

One doesn't have to be the loneliest number—embrace time alone. It is important to find people with whom you can connect. But, even more important is learning to be at peace with yourself. Relationships take spending time together to learn about each other. Your relationship with yourself is no different. If you want to find personal fulfillment, you are going to have to get comfortable being alone. My good friend and fitness trainer, Pamela, calls it her "sit and stare time." It is the time when you carve out a few hours or a few days just to be alone. Go for a drive, sit on the patio with a cup of coffee, reflect on the things you are discovering about yourself, talk to God about them. The Bible tells us, "He is closer than a brother." You can tell Him anything. Time alone will help you feel comfortable with the real you. Embrace the essence of who you really are, and then you will be well-equipped to share yourself with others.

Reach Out. Giving your time and energy to enrich the lives of others will do more to uncover your soul than anything else you can do. In a recent devotional, I read about a lady who wanted to start a pet grooming business, but she didn't have the money she needed to advertise. She went to her local animal shelter and volunteered to groom the pets to help increase their chances for adoption. Interestingly, the harder she worked, the more her own business grew by word of mouth. Finally, she ended up with more clients than she could handle. God tells us in Proverbs 11:24-25, "Be stingy and lose everything, the generous … prosper." If you have a need in your life, stop dwelling on it. Instead, get out there and help meet a need you see in the life of another. If you need a job, volunteer at your child's school while you're looking for work. If you're praying for God to bless your business, focus on providing the best service possible to the clients you do have and ask God to prosper them. The Bible says when you "Give generously…your gifts will return to you later."

Enjoy. If you've examined your life and aren't happy with what you see, maybe all you need is to change your vantage point. Practice looking at the good things in your life. Find something to enjoy in every minute of every day. Don't worry—at first you won't be very good at it, but you'll get better with practice—and it will change your life.

In 2001, when H-E-B Grocery Company recruited me to San Antonio, Texas, to be their Culinary Manager, my son, Jay, was a junior in high school. Jay is the youngest of my four children and the only boy. I was hesitant to relocate when Jay had so many good friends and was so plugged in to school and church in Lubbock. I turned H-E-B down on the job offer a couple of times, but the company was persistent. When I finally discussed the possibility with Jay, to my surprise he saw the move as an opportunity to expand his horizons. All my other children were in college, so Jay and I relocated, just the two of us. It could have been a difficult move. We had to adjust to life in the city, the traffic, long commutes, and the anonymity (I had been in Lubbock for 26 years, and Jay had lived there his entire life, so everywhere we went we knew tons of people. In San Antonio we knew no one.) But, when we decided to make the move, we agreed it would be the "Jan & Jay Adventure." We were determined to focus on the good things and do what we could to make our adventure fun and exciting.

In hindsight, the move was the best thing we ever did. It was a new beginning. One of the first things we did to make the move fun was to start fresh. We were accustomed to living on a dime in Lubbock. All the furniture we had was, shall we say, "well-loved?" When we moved, we sold the house and practically everything in it. We bought a new house on a half-acre outside of San Antonio in the Hill Country. It was in a beautiful area, and coming from the flat lands of Lubbock, we thought it was especially beautiful. We shopped together for furniture and had great fun making our new home look like a Hill Country retreat.

Of course, the demands of school and tennis for Jay and the new job for me made finding time together to share our "Jan & Jay Adventure" more challenging. The one thing we held sacred was meeting at the house in the evenings to make dinner together. After dinner, we would go for a walk down to the end of our road to watch the sun set over the hills. Often Jay would bring friends along for dinner. It gave me a great chance to meet his new friends and find out what exciting things were going on in his life. One of the greatest honors I had during our adventure was his prom night. He and three friends asked if I would prepare a gourmet meal for them and their dates prior to the prom. I had so much fun pulling out the china and crystal and really making a special meal for them. If you have teenagers, you know it is quite an honor to be asked to be a part of their lives, and I tried to enjoy every minute of it. I firmly believe that making the decision to enjoy the move, and the new experiences that came our way, helped create one of the most treasured times of my life. Jay and I will always have the amazing memories of our days in the Hill Country.

By getting to the C.O.R.E. of the matter, you will be fulfilled in ways you might have never dreamed possible.

By connecting with God and with others, learning to embrace alone time, reaching out to share yourself with others, and making a conscious effort to enjoy life, you will have learned the secret to building a strong personal core. You have a choice in life; you can choose to endure each day doing the minimal amount necessary to make it through, or you can grab life by the horns and become all you were created to be.

"But they that wait upon the Lord shall renew their strength; they shall mount up with wings as eagles; they shall run and not be weary; and they shall walk and not faint."

ISAIAH 40:31

As you grow to embrace the idea of getting your second wind many of you will endeavor to adopt a life of healthy eating and physical activity. I want to challenge you to be among the few who learn to soar. Get in touch with your core. Discover your potential. Find out who you are and explore the opportunities of becoming all God created you to be. Release your spirit to soar to new heights. It is a quest that will not disappoint—it can be the difference between a good life and a great one.

CHAPTER 10

You Are Who You Are

If we are honest with ourselves, most of us will admit one of our greatest fears is to be seen in our most real, vulnerable state. We much prefer to have our makeup on, our hair done, our houses picked up, when company drops by. We strive to be considered top in our profession, of highest value as an employee, the best mom, the most beautiful wife ... and the list goes on and on. These labels are how we perceive our value as a person. But, we can't all be the best at everything. It's impossible. God created some of us with natural athletic ability, some with academic prowess, some with flawless skin and silky beautiful hair, but no one can have it all. For those who fall into the category of perfectionist, this is a difficult concept to grasp. If we have hundreds of stellar qualities and just a few where others are superior, we agonize over how to improve—and if we can't improve, then we try desperately to hide our inferiority.

I'll give you an example. I am married to a fabulous tennis player. We belong to a great club where he plays, and at that club most all the wives play equally as well, if not better, than their husbands. All the women were inviting me to play on their team, assuming that because Bruce plays well, that I would, too. Well, I played one season, and quite honestly,

I am terrible at tennis. I have good endurance in the heat because I am a distance runner, but I have no hand-eye co-ordination. I've taken lessons and played in clinics; I've gone to the courts alone and hit untold millions of serves trying to improve.

I fake it well. On the surface, I look like a tennis player. I have all the right little tennis outfits. I have a great racket, tennis shoes, and a really cute tennis bag my kids got me for my birthday. It's when I hit the court that I can no longer pretend. Every week at practice, I would just cringe to go out on the court with the team and let everyone actually see how bad I am at tennis. After I finally finished that one league season, I have not returned. When they get desperate for a substitute, they call me, but I still have not gone back. Why? Because I hate the humiliation I feel at not being a competent player. Plus, I know Bruce would love it if I were a great player. We would have so much fun playing mixed doubles together, and I hate that I disappoint him. Not that he puts any pressure on me. He is fine with me being exactly who I am, but I put tons of pressure on myself to be amazing at everything.

I'm trying to get better at this and I think I'm progressing. Accepting yourself as you are is one of the most wonderful things I've found so far about growing older. I have discovered that I can let go of my need to be perfect and accept things about myself that drove me crazy when I was younger. An example some of you may be able to identify with: I've had four kids, one by C-section and a hysterectomy that was done back in the day when the norm was to make the incision from one side to the other, severing all your stomach muscles. I used to spend a lot of time working out, going to aerobics classes, running, lifting weights, trying to get rid of my little belly. I hate it. It has been just in the last few years that I've been able to take a step back and say, "I've worked hard to earn this body. I've birthed four fabulous children that have blessed my life beyond measure. I may not ever have a totally flat belly again, like I did 30 years ago, but, you know what, that is okay. I have a strong, healthy body and that is all that truly matters."

One of the most important gifts you can give yourself as you age is to accept, and even embrace, the real you. There is nothing as wonderful as spending time with someone who has mastered the art of loving themselves just as they are. The walls are down, the pretense is gone, and what you see is what you get. We all know people who embody this trait, and they are probably the people you most enjoy spending time. Perhaps it's your crazy aunt who can be found every Tuesday morning playing hymns and singing off key at the top of her lungs with a group of seniors at the assisted living center. Maybe it is a favorite retired friend who has just discovered her inner athlete. She now loves road racing. She dresses her old, less than perfect body in brightly colored running gear and proudly runs her 12-minute mile all the way to the finish line. She is famous for her finish-line celebrations that closely resemble the victory dance of the first finishing female at the Boston Marathon. These people are so much fun to be around because they've learned to "love the skin they're in." Their lives are no longer filled with pretense and barriers. They have learned to accept themselves for who they are, and it has freed their spirit to celebrate life.

Accepting yourself as you are is not an excuse to stop trying to improve. Remember, I'm writing this book to encourage you to be the best you can be. I want to help you see the person God created you to be, the beautiful things about you and the things you'd rather change about yourself. Blended together, all of this uniquely equips you to fulfill the plan God has for your life.

I love this verse in Philippians; it is a great source of encouragement for me to keep striving:

I don't mean to say I am perfect. I haven't
learned all I should even yet,
but I keep working toward that day
when I will be all that Christ saved me for
and wants me to be.

No.... I am still not all I should be
but I am bringing all my energies to bear on this one
    thing:
forgetting the past
looking forward to what lies ahead,
I strain to reach the end of the race
and receive the prize...

PHILIPPIANS 3:12-13

The message in this chapter is this: You have some amazing gifts, some things you are good at, things you excel at. You also have some things about your body or your personality, or your circumstances, that you would love to change if you could. To age graciously, you've got to learn to pray the same prayer St. Francis of Assisi did:

"Lord grant me the serenity to accept the things I cannot
change, the courage to change the things I can, and the
wisdom to know the difference."

It is a prayer you've heard all your life, but read it again and truly let your spirit absorb its powerful message. Learning to accept yourself is tough enough, but learning to "bloom where you are planted" can be an even greater challenge. I can't explain why bad things happen to good people or why it seems some of us must deal with more difficult circumstances than others. I do know we all struggle. At least I know that in my head, but when I'm going through a tough time and I'm lying awake staring at the ceiling in the middle of the night, I sometimes feel like I am the only person in the world with struggles. I look out at my friends, my associates, my competitors, and it seems they don't have a care in the world. Isn't it funny how the grass is always greener in someone else's backyard?

Being in the counseling field, I will tell you, I've had beautiful, wealthy clients who walk in looking like they have the world by the tail, but as we talk, I find they have crumbling marriages, terminal illnesses they are dealing with, or multiple other life struggles. Once they let you in close enough to peek inside their world, the little cracks begin to show, and you can see we all have issues, situations and circumstances to deal with.

I have a book I received as a high school graduation gift. It is a little book entitled *Yes* by Ann Kiemel that I've read hundreds of times. I've used it to teach Bible study classes. I've marked all over it. I've shared it with numerous friends and colleagues who were going through personal struggles. I am a nutrition consultant for a few assisted-living centers in South Texas and on this particular night I was in Rockport, Texas. I brought the book with me and had been out on a lawn chair watching the waves hit the coastline and rereading the book once again.

I find such inspiration in Ann's writing. It is simple, almost prose-like, and easy to read. It talks about saying "Yes" to Jesus no matter what he asks you to do. Ann talks in the book about her longing to have a spectacular life story like Mother Theresa or Martin Luther King Jr., and then finally coming to the understanding that God has simply called her to live for Him in her own neighborhood. It's the same calling most of us have. It's not glamorous and certainly most of the time it's not that exciting, but it is real. And when we allow God to take our reality and use it for His glory, miraculous things begin to happen in the lives of the people we come in contact. Here is how Ann describes God's desire for her life. I would encourage you to read her words replacing Ann's name with your own.

> "Ann, My will for you is that you be whole.
> that you keep Me Lord of your total being.
> that you learn to be content and happy in every
> situation. be a servant at all times ... with joy.
> learn to cook more in the kitchen.
> take long walks and feel Me in the air and wide
> sky and stretching skyline and noises of people.
>
> Ann, I desire that you will be poised.
> your heart steady and determined to face each
> morning with courage and good will.
> I want you to move through life with utter
> confidence in who you are: MINE ...
> and where you are going: out to the hurting.
> lonely, wide world around you ...
> taking love and heart and wonder and warmth
> and the Song of Jesus ...
> dream impossible dreams, but build them into the
> normal life you lead.
> make every day incredible just by what you exude
> in your eyes and handshake and easy spirit.
> be self-contained in Me."

Jesus simply asks us to accept who we are in Him and make the very most of every day we are given. This kind of self-acceptance is simple, but it is certainly not easy. (I learned that saying from my tennis coach—he would tell me a good serve is *simple*—you toss the ball up and hit it over the net into the little green square, but it is not easy to learn how to do that—as I can attest.) Well, it is the same with learning to accept yourself just as you are. We so often use crutches to cope with our shortcomings and feelings of personal inadequacy. Drinking, drugs, illicit sex, gossip, anger, greed—all are a means of dealing with our feelings of not quite measuring up to expectations—either those we have of ourselves or those we perceive others to have of us.

To find the joy, contentment, and fulfillment you long for as you learn to live in the reality of who you are, you will need to find a way to come to terms with "loving the skin you're in."

In true David Letterman style, the:

Top 10 Things You Need To Know About Getting Real:

10: **Being "real" means spending some time alone with yourself to discover the "real" you.** Many of us have spent years covering up our real self to please others. It may take some alone time to peel away the layers to discover for yourself what it means to be authentically you."

9: **Being "real" is not an excuse for being sloppy.** Some use it as an excuse for "letting it all hang out" when, in reality, they are short on manners and consideration for the feelings of others. They are the crass, offensive people you know who say things like, "Hey, this is just who I am; I can't help it," when they say unkind words to hurt someone.

8: **Being "real" means taking personal responsibility for who you are and what your life will stand for.** It means taking care of your physical body, your mind, and your soul. Determine what that means for you, then commit to obedience in that lifestyle. Your personal style can take on many different looks. Maybe taking care of yourself is becoming vegetarian, or practicing yoga, or growing fruits and vegetables in your own garden, or training for a triathlon or walking your dog every evening after dinner. Whatever you deem important, commit to following through to the best of your ability.

7: **Being "real" is your legacy; a priceless gift you can give to your family.** What better example can we give to our kids than to be true to who we really are? They will see from your example that when you do what you love and are true to the things about which you are passionate, the roller coaster of life will be full of joy and excitement.

6: **Being "real" frees your spirit to soar to new heights.** It allows you to explore the entire person God created you to be. When we try to live to please others, life is hard. Making life choices, such as choosing a career or a spouse, can seem overwhelming. But when you free yourself to be real, your life pieces fit together much more easily, thus allowing you to become all you were meant to be.

5: **Being "real" means letting go of seeking approval from others.** When you can find contentment in who you are, you no longer need the approval of others to be okay. By accepting yourself, with all your quirky little behaviors, likes and dislikes, personality traits and passions, you free yourself to enter a world of confidence like you've never known.

People—boyfriends, girlfriends, employers, family and friends—will see you in a completely different light and will be drawn to your confident spirit because you have dared to value yourself regardless of what others might think of you.

4: **Being "real" means embracing your weaknesses.** Accept yourself by acknowledging the things at which you are good, and accept the things at which you are not so good. A good friend of mine gave me a great piece of advice when I opened my own business. He said, "Do what you do best, and hire the rest." It has proven to be sage wisdom. I am a visionary. I like to paint the big picture. I get really bogged down in the little (but very important) things like billing and dealing with insurance companies. The first thing I did was hire a business office manager who handles the details for me, and it has made all the difference in the success of my company.

3: **Being "real" means drawing wisdom from past experiences and moving confidently into your future.** Most all of us have made some major life-shattering mistakes. Don't hide from them; learn from them. It is never too late to turn around and start moving toward health and well-being.

2: **Being "real" means being true to yourself.** It means not compromising what is important to you. It means discovering your "non-negotiables"—those things you will not bend on, no matter what. Do you remember the story of Elisabeth Elliot? She and her husband, Jim, were missionaries to the Auca Indians in Ecuador. Jim was killed trying to take the good news of Jesus Christ to this tribe. Even after the violent death of her husband, she continued working with the Indians in Ecuador. Forgiveness and her unwavering dedication to missions allowed her to stand firm in the face of unbelievable personal pain and hardship. Most of us will never have to face such severe trials, but we do face little opportunities each day where we have a choice—will we choose to be faithful to our core values, or will we take the easy way out?

1: Being "real" means honoring and respecting the individualism in others while still being true to yourself.

*For what does it profit a man to gain the whole world,
and forfeit his soul?*

MARK 8:36

Discovering who you are and accepting yourself as you are—the good, the bad, and the ugly—makes life rich and meaningful, but if we do it at the expense of those we love, we will be left with nothing. The most important things in life are the relationships we form with our families and friends. As you are spending time to find out who you are, make sure you apply the same rules to others. Give them the freedom to be themselves, just as you are demanding the freedom to be you.

Nothing brings this message home like a visit with family during the holidays. Vacations spent with families can be some of the most stressful days of the year. Much of this stress relates to the fact we are trying to break free of the labels and expectations we perceive that have been placed on us by our families. While on our own, in our own cities, living our own lives, it is easier to be real, but when we get back in that family environment, we often revert to the labels our families put on us as kids.

Breaking free from your past does not have to be a huge family drama. As you find who you are and begin to accept yourself, you will find a wonderful self-confidence that comes from being real. When you return home to spend time with your family, be "matter-of-factly" you, walking into family situations with poise and confidence in whom you are. You may be surprised to find this is just the push your family needs to begin to treat you with the respect you deserve.

I think this is an especially sensitive area for mothers and daughters, or maybe it seems that way since that is the relationship I am most familiar with. Since I have a mother and three daughters, I am going to try to be brave enough to broach this subject. I spent a lot of years trying to measure up to what I thought my mom wanted me to be. (Don't we all?)

My situation was unique because in my mind, my mom is perfect, so the reality was I had no chance. I never saw her angry, moody, sweaty, tired, or unprepared for anything. You think I am exaggerating, but I am not. I still remember one morning when I was in elementary school; she was making biscuits for my brother and me for breakfast. She was baking them on a non-stick pan and when she pulled them out of the oven, they slid off the pan and onto the floor. I remember her leaving the room, crying. That is one of the only times I can remember her even remotely losing it.

As I started my family, this was my "picture" of what I was supposed to be like. However, remember I am, by nature, much more like my father, so when I drop biscuits, it is not a calm reaction. I am likely to stomp and scream. It took me many years to come to grips with the fact that I can be like that and still be okay. I get angry. I get mad. I get disappointed. I get tired. I get in bad moods. I get confrontational. I am not always a lady. I love to work hard in my yard. I love to run. I love to sweat, and that is okay. My favorite days are spent putting on my running clothes, pulling my hair back in a ponytail, and not wearing makeup. I've hardly ever seen my mom without her makeup. She gets up early and is "fixed up" before anyone else in the house is awake.

So here is the point. I had to learn that it was okay for me to not be as perfect as my mom. Then, perhaps even more important, I had to learn it was okay for her to be who she is. To me, that was the biggest lesson of all.

Of course, there is that whole mother-daughter thing from the other side of the coin. I am a mother of three wonderful young adult daughters. And, they don't tell me, but I know they perceive my "comments" about their lifestyles, life choices, boyfriends, careers, what they eat, how they wear their hair, the clothes that they wear, and on and on—I know they think they are not measuring up to my expectations.

They know I place a lot of value on health and they think I am disappointed if they eat junk and choose not to make fitness a part of their lifestyle. Part of it is that we moms have trouble knowing when to quit "mothering" and when to start enjoying the company of our adult children. I want them to be healthy and look and feel their very best, so I probably let my passion on that subject surface too often. But, in fairness to all the mothers out there—part of it is just us interacting, making conversation in an attempt to maintain a relationship with adult children who are leaving home to build their own lives.

Regardless, we have to acknowledge the power the mother-daughter relationship holds in our lives. Our love and concern can very often be misconstrued by our daughters as meddling. The key is learning when to hold fast and when to let go. We love our children so much that we often want to hold on too tight—even after it is time to let them soar.

My father spoke at my high school graduation ceremony.

In his speech, he used a quote by Robert A. Raines that so beautifully depicts the evolution of our relationship with our children as they grow into adulthood.

"He who would bind to himself a joy,
Doth the winged life destroy,
But he that kisses the joy as it flies
Lives in eternity's sunrise."

As you learn to accept yourself for who you are, make sure you learn to allow others to be who God created them to be, as well. This acceptance of the differences of others goes not just for mothers and daughters, but for all of life's relationships. You are who you are, and they are who they are. Quit trying to change people into who you'd like them to be. When you can learn to accept and enjoy the person God created you to be and when you can extend that freedom to those you love, you will find peace and joy in your relationships like you never knew possible.

CHAPTER 11

Finish Strong

The decision to get your second wind is the starting point in your search to add purpose and meaning to your life. As we've explored in this book, one of the greatest challenges is taking the first step. Once you get started, there is a renaissance phase where you recreate yourself into a healthy, well-balanced person. Each step on your personal path to wellness must be taken and plays a key role as you reinvent yourself. You have made the decision to take charge of your life and courageously walk the steps toward health, now comes the endurance race. The excitement of discovering new things about yourself and making changes that bring dramatic results in your health and well-being is exhilarating. Now comes the day to day practice of all that you have learned. As any professional marathoner will tell you, crossing the finish line in victory is the best feeling, but one that they work day in and day out for, and may only experience a few times in their career. How do we keep the stamina and the determination to finish strong?

Remember when you were little and your parents would say "Don't start something you can't finish." It is a really great lesson, and it takes some of us longer than others to embrace the idea. What they really were trying to teach you was to "finish strong." The discipline to complete what you have set out to do is the secret to success. I've watched my husband on the tennis court. Even when he is down, he never gives up. He never lets down. He powers through to complete the match and often his determination is the difference between defeat and victory in the match.

As you embark on life's journey, the difference between mediocrity and success is how determined you are to finish strong. Often when I am running a long race, and I'm tired, and my legs hurt, and I just want to slow down or stop, I repeat these words to myself, "Finish strong, Jan." It reminds me that I am living for more than immediate pleasure and gratification, that my goals and my life are about the bigger picture. Success does not mean you will never fail. Rather, it is dedicating yourself to being the very best you can be—in everything you do every day. An unwavering commitment to finish strong will reflect in how you feed and train your body, how you relate to the people in your life, how you approach your career, how you face obstacles, and ultimately how you face death.

What are some ways you can train yourself to stay focused on the task at hand and finish strong? Here are four life lessons we all should learn about the rewards of finishing what you start:

Life Lesson No. 1: Finish Healthy

I am horrified at the state of health in which we find our nation, and I am convinced we have each contributed by making a cumulative series of bad choices in diet and exercise. The only way out of this mess is that we as a nation, as families, and as individuals must plan to be successful by determining to have the willpower to make wise choices. We have numerous opportunities each day to be successful:

- Will I set my alarm to get up and work out before work, or turn it off and sleep in?

- Will I choose a healthy breakfast full of whole grains, fruit, protein and low-fat dairy, or will I stop by for a sausage and egg biscuit with hash browns?

- Will I choose a healthy lunch or give in and go with the group from the office going out for enchiladas?

- Will I plan for healthy meals and take time to shop for what I need on the weekend, or will I take the easy way out and stop by for a pizza on the way home from work?

- Will I make the choice to be active when I get home, or will I flop down on the sofa until I drag myself in to raid the fridge?

- Will I choose a big bowl of ice cream and cookies for my after-dinner treat, or will I choose a bowl of fresh berries with low-fat yogurt?

These are just a handful of the daily scenarios we face. Being healthy requires making a conscious decision to do what's best for our bodies. If you choose the easy path, the path that follows the motto, "If it feels good, do it," you will reap the consequences of that lifestyle as you age, and believe me, it is not pretty.

As a dietitian, I counsel people in a variety of phases and stages of life. I see young children to elderly adults and everyone in between. A few months ago, I was visiting with a 27-year-old patient who weighed in at our initial visit at more than 200 pounds. More alarming is that she has an 8-year-old nephew who lives with her who weighs 180 pounds. As she was telling me about the habit they had gotten into of having fast food delivered to their door and sitting in front of the television to play video games for the evening, I reminded her of the importance of making wise choices every moment of every day. Every choice counts—it either takes you farther down the path to health and wellness or it will take you down the path to your demise. I am happy to tell you that they have made some changes and are beginning to see the results of making healthier choices. She has joined a gym. They go together to the park close to their home several evenings a week, and she is trying her hand at what I call "assembly cooking"—buying healthy convenience items at the store to serve for dinner. She has lost close to twenty pounds, her nephew is growing taller and has lost a couple of pounds, and they are enjoying spending quality time together as a family.

The childhood obesity epidemic we face is wrecking the health of our youth. As parents and concerned adults, we must model a healthy lifestyle. We must light the way to health and wellness through making wise choices in what we eat and in our willingness to get up off the sofa and get active. By demonstrating healthy choices and providing an avenue for our children to eat well and be active, we are setting an example for our children to know how to be healthy.

Consulting for nursing homes makes me even more passionate about the importance of making good choices. I see patients not much older than I who have abused their bodies by overindulging in food and drink and refusing to recognize the value of exercise, and it has left them old beyond their years. Often they are suffering from uncontrolled type 2 diabetes, which can result in peripheral vascular disease, which leads to blindness, amputations, kidney failure and heart disease. Now they are in a wheelchair or bedridden in a nursing home unable to take care of themselves. All of this pain and heartache because one day in their youth, they decided to indulge themselves, and they never found the willpower or self-discipline to stop. It can be as innocuous as choosing to super-size a fast-food order or deciding that lying on the sofa watching TV is easier than lacing up tennis shoes. We all do this occasionally, but when it becomes a lifestyle, we are putting ourselves at great risk for chronic disease.

Newsflash: Whether you are 8 or 80, health takes discipline.

Good health requires that we find the courage to take the road less traveled. If our children's friends are eating bags of chips and playing hours of video games, we must teach them how to dare to be different. If our friends are leaving work to go straight to "happy hour" in the evening, or if they think sweating isn't ladylike, then we must be strong enough to go it alone and get active. We must know how to make healthy choices … and then make them.

If you have made a series of bad choices, the good news is it is never too late to change. I'm not promising you can reverse all the damage you have done, but I do know that by determining from this point forward to practice a healthy lifestyle, you can be successful. You can improve your energy level, take control of chronic health issues you are facing, and actually enjoy life again. Take my 27-year-old client and her nephew. They are now on the path to recovery. We've discussed a plan for how they can be successful and they are taking the necessary steps to get there. They now *know how* to get back on track; it's up to them to make the hard choices every day *to live the change.*

Life Lesson No.2: Finish with Honor

Honor is a word we speak very little, but it has such power. I've thought a lot about that word, and I think it is such a foreign concept to most of us that we have trouble defining it. The odd thing is, we know it when we see it. A person of honor is a person of character. Not all successful people are honorable, and it seems success without character is empty. Think of those you know who have achieved financial success and notoriety without strong character to back it up. When this happens it is a natural instinct to try to fill the void with something. Our celebrity heroes often turn to sex, alcohol, and drugs to make their success "taste" better. But, as longtime Penn State football coach, Joe Paterno so aptly describes in his famous quote:

> *"Success without honor is an unseasoned dish; it will satisfy your hunger, but it won't taste good."*
>
> —JOE PATERNO

Honor is not something you are born with; each of us has to develop it on our own. You may have been born into a family with strong character and moral values, but you will still have to build your own personal legacy. To be successful and finish strong you must create your own code of honor. It is a code you live by no matter what comes your way. It is a code that carries you through tough times, sustains you through the routine, and helps you soar through the good times in your life.

I want to challenge you to seek a life based on honor. The success you achieve will be sweeter and your life will have purpose and meaning. You will find designing your own personal code of honor to be instrumental in guiding you to success. The key is taking the time to map your plan. I encourage you to write it down and put it in your wallet or desk drawer where you can look at it often. By taking time to review and practice it, your code will move from head knowledge to heart knowledge. It will become your creed—the rules you live by. You will be known for these traits among your friends and family members. This is your chance to leave a legacy of one who lived an honorable life. Here is a template to get you started:

My Personal Code of Honor

1. **I will honor my body.** You are in control of your body. You decide how to feed and exercise it. Mary McCord, a friend and fitness instructor, tells her clients to think of their body as their closest friend.

> *"You have a friend who has been with you from the time you drew your very first breath and who will be with you until you breathe your very last. This friend has stuck by you through thick and thin. When you've accomplished great things it has done everything possible to help you do your very best. When you have fallen, it has picked you back up and helped you back to wholeness. Even when you treat it poorly, it tries very hard to overcome the mistreatment and be the very best it can be. We get one chance to walk through life with this loyal friend, our body. Treat it with respect and it will be the foundation on which you build greatness."*

How do you honor such a trusted friend? Begin with making small, wise choices and work up to bigger challenges. Here are a few ideas to get you started:

  a. Commit to eating breakfast every day.

b. Commit to stop eating before you are stuffed.

c. Commit to choosing nutrient-rich foods—no junk.

d. Commit to getting 30 minutes of exercise every day.

e. Commit to 30 minutes of strength training three days a week.

f. Commit to doing what it takes to stay within 10 percent of your ideal body weight.

g. Commit to getting at least eight hours of sleep every night.

Changes I will make to get started in the right direction:

_____

_____

_____

_____

_____

2. **I will honor my husband/wife.** You will be amazed at the change in your relationship with your spouse as you choose to treat yourself and your partner with respect. So often, through years of marriage we can get into bad habits. Both are at fault—one spouse treats the other as if they were the lesser half, and their partner tolerates it. Here is the great thing about honor. You honor yourself

and command respect. You honor your spouse and show them respect. It's God's way and it works.

a. **Let your speech be kind**. Have you ever really listened to your tone when you talk to your spouse? You will get much better results if you speak kindly.

b. **Do something special**. It doesn't have to be big, just something to show you know what is important to them and that you care—maybe take time to cook or go out for a meal they really enjoy, or go watch them play a sport they are involved in, or clean their car. The key here is you do something nice for them and treat them with respect, but you also honor and care for yourself, and do not allow them to abuse your kindness—I am not advocating blind servanthood. When they notice the change (and they will), communicate your needs and your desire for the relationship to grow into a mutually caring, loving relationship where you each feel safe, loved, and truly happy to be together.

Changes I can make to begin showing more respect to my spouse:

_____

_____

_____

_____

_____

3. **I will honor my family**. When I am visiting with clients, I hear many references to family members. Often they are blamed for weight issues and our inability to cope with life. Obviously, some truth exists in what they are telling me—they did not see a good example modeled for them. The cool thing is this: as you grow more comfortable with who you are, you move from looking for people to blame for your shortcomings, and you begin to take responsibility for overcoming them.

Changes I can make to demonstrate honor toward my family members:

_____

_____

_____

_____

_____

_____

4. **I will honor my employer**. Your employer has entrusted you with a responsibility in their company. I will tell you as a business owner, that company is their "baby." They have invested greatly in it, both personally and financially, and they have chosen you to participate with them to achieve great things. You need to honor that trust by doing your very best.

Changes I can make to show my boss I respect and honor his/her leadership in my life:

_____

_____

_____

_____

_____

_____

5. I will honor my employees and/or co-workers. By the same token, employers need to recognize the people they've hired to be a part of their company are dedicated to making their dreams become reality. Employees work incredibly hard and should be treated with honor and respect. Find ways to show them how much they are appreciated. Your co-workers are individuals you spend a lot of time with. It is important you build relationships with them based on mutual respect.

Changes I can make at work that will show my employees or co-workers I respect their efforts:

_____

_____

_____

_____

_____

_____

6. **I will honor my community.** The community where you live is your responsibility. If you are a success but have done nothing to make your little corner of the world a better place to be, then what have you really accomplished? Plan to make a difference.

Changes I can make toward becoming more involved in my community:

_____

_____

_____

_____

_____

7. **I will honor God.** You have been given talents and treasures to use to glorify God. As you use those gifts and find success, make sure you give credit to the One who blessed you with the abilities and the wisdom to do great things.

Changes I can make toward giving God the honor and glory He deserves in my life:

_____

_____

_____

_____

_____

*"When I stand before God at the end of my life, I would
hope that I would not have a single bit of talent left, and
could say, 'I used everything you gave me.'"*

ERMA BOMBECK

Life Lesson No.3: Finish with Dignity.

Being successful doesn't always mean things go your way or that you always get the results you desire. Sometimes it means accepting the reality of your life with grace and courage. We all have tragedy and adversity that comes our way. How we deal with hurt and disappointment reveals our true character and that speaks volumes to those watching us from the sidelines. No matter who you are, you have people close to you and those you don't even know who are waiting to see how you will respond to the obstacles and challenges that come your way.

When I think about finishing strong, I think of my father. He was in the hospital for cancer treatment when he began going into heart failure. He was placed on a ventilator in the intensive care unit, and we, as a family, were faced with a difficult decision. He had made it clear to us that he did not want his life prolonged by being placed on life support. His body was riddled with cancer. He had fought a long, painful fight against this insidious disease, and now it was time to let him go. Tearfully, prayerfully, in a most holy moment, my mom, my brother and I all gathered in the room to tell him goodbye. We stood there as they disconnected all the tubes. His breathing slowed, and with his last ounce of strength, he smiled and said "I'm going to miss you guys." We stood beside his bed to be with him as he passed from our arms into the arms of Jesus. I remember my brother starting to recite my dad's favorite poem "I met God in the morning when my day was at its best." My mom and I joined in. Then, we quietly, reverently sang "Amazing Grace."

When we've been there ten thousand years
Bright shining as the sun
There's no less days
To sing God's praise
Than when we first begun …

… and he was gone. We stepped out from behind the curtain to leave, and his nurse was crying. She commented to us that being an ICU nurse, she deals with death almost every day. She sees families in agony at the loss of their loved one, but she was moved to tears to watch as we were able to pull together as a family to help my father maintain his dignity, and finish strong.

Some of our greatest successes in this life will come when we can muddle through the challenges of life, holding onto each other and our faith for strength. People are watching you. They are rooting for you. Our hearts are warmed and our faith in humanity is renewed when we witness those who overcome adversity to finish strong.

Therefore, since we have so great a cloud of witnesses
surrounding us, let us also lay aside every encumbrance
and the sin which so easily entangles us, and let us run
with endurance the race that is set before us.
Hebrews 12:1

Life Lesson No. 4: Finishing with Determination.

The determining factor in competitions where opponents are fairly matched boils down to who is mentally tough enough to stay focused on the goal until the very end. You have to be passionate in your desire to finish strong. You have to believe you are capable of winning and refuse to settle for anything less than victory. Life is a challenge—that means you will face obstacles. Success comes when you learn how to use your obstacles as building blocks.

"A successful man is one who can lay a firm foundation with the bricks others have thrown at him."
—DAVID BRINKLEY

My oldest daughter, Leigh, has always been an amazing athlete. As a senior in high school, with strong urging from the track coach, she joined the track team. She had never participated in track before, but that year, she went to state and won third in the 5,000-meter race. She was offered a track scholarship to Texas Tech University and competed as a Red Raider her entire college career.

In 1999, her junior year of college, she had become a truly outstanding competitor. She was winning every race she entered. She was chosen to go to Spain to represent the USA in the World University Games which she won handily in a field of awesome competitors. As incredible as this and all her other accolades were, there is one race that stands out far above the rest.

It was in 1999 at the NCAA Track & Field Championships in Boise, Idaho. It was the last race of the evening, the 10,000-meter race. Her father and I had both made the trip to watch her compete. It was a perfect evening, and Leigh started the race as the clear favorite to win. As you can imagine, we were nervous—as all parents are sitting in the stands watching their child compete at that level, but we knew she had a very good shot to win.

If you've ever seen a distance race like this begin, you

know that when the start gun sounds, the field is crowded with runners. It takes a few laps for them to find their pace and begin to spread out. As Leigh began the second lap, I saw her motion to her coach, and I could see something was not right. I couldn't believe my eyes. She ran another lap obviously under duress. When she rounded the stadium again, I could see her coach telling her to stop and put her shoe back on. In the crowd of runners, someone had stepped on the back of Leigh's shoe and pulled it off her heel. She had been running the last lap with her toes barely hanging on to her shoe. Her coach was motioning her to stop and slip it back onto her heel. What he didn't know is that Leigh had double knotted her shoe to help prevent this very thing from happening. Much to her coach's horror, rather than stopping for a second to slip it back on, she knelt down on the track, untied the knots, put her shoe back on, retied it, and got up to start again. By this time the last runners had long passed her by, and she was a good half-lap behind even the slowest runners. Her coach, her father, and I and the entire packed stadium at Boise State sat in stunned silence.

Leigh had trained diligently for this race, and she had a plan in place to win it. Knowing she had 23 laps to go, she knew better than to race to catch up with the crowd. That would leave her exhausted and unable to finish. She resumed the pace she had planned for, and her coach gave her splits from the sidelines to try to get her back into the race. Slowly, confidently, she began to catch some of the girls. She passed a few and continued to run her race. She passed a few more, and by this time, the crowd was beginning to acknowledge she might still have a chance. With just a few laps to go, she caught up to the third-place runner. She continued to press on, and within a couple of laps, she was running neck and neck with the second-place competitor. At this point all of the people in the stadium was on their feet cheering the little girl from Texas Tech who lost her shoe, but still found the courage to stay in the race. With the bell lap to go, Leigh began her kick to the finish. The leader was a brilliant runner from Notre Dame and she was a good eight to ten strides ahead. Leigh stayed behind her and then with about a quarter-lap to go, she passed her. At this point, the crowd was going crazy, and my heart was beating out of my chest.

Leigh Daniel came from behind and won the 10,000-meter NCAA Championships.

Afterward, when one of the announcers asked how she was able to stay in the race, both mentally and physically, she said, "I was not going to let a shoe stand between me and my dream." That is the definition of what it means to finish strong. Leigh had a dream and she had trained diligently to prepare herself for victory. In spite of seemingly insurmountable odds, she did not let anything stand in the way of her success.

Isn't that how it is in life? We must discipline ourselves to overcome circumstances and challenges that try to stand in the way of our dreams. True success is not handed to us on a silver platter; it is claimed in spite of hardship and adversity.

Finishing strong is about living a life of courage—the courage to make wise decisions, the courage to stand for something, the courage to live a life of honor and integrity no matter what obstacles or hardships come your way. It is about living a healthy, happy life using the wisdom you've gained from all the earlier accomplishments and mistakes you've made. Let those lessons empower you. Dig deep within your soul to learn who you really are and where you are going. Commit yourself to excellence in all things—big and small. Find the courage to start again when you fall down. Find the perseverance you need to walk through trials. And, most important, find the determination you need to never, ever give up.

Finish strong.

Bibliography

1. **Honoring & Identifying Your True Hunger Chart.**
   http://www.move.va.gov/download/NewHandouts/Nutrition/N04_HungerAndFullness.pdf MOVE! Weight
   Management Program. 18 April 2007. VA National
   Center for Health Promotion and Disease Prevention
   http://www.move.va.gov/

2. **Fad Diet Cycle Graph.** Losing Weight. 8 August 2007.
   A.D.A.M. <http://www.medhelp.org/>

3. **Calorie Meal Plan Exchanges.** This is a general information chart that varies depending on professional opinions.

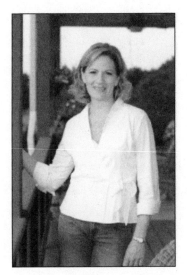

About the Author

Jan Tilley is president of Jan Tilley & Associates, Inc., a nutrition marketing and consulting firm promoting healthy living through nutrition and fitness. Tilley has more than twenty years of experience in the food and nutrition industry. She is a registered dietician and has an MS in nutrition from Texas Tech University.